THE WAY TO INFINITE HEALTH

YULIA LILITH ROSE

Disclaimer

This book is designed for educational purposes only and is not intended to serve as medical advice. The information provided in this book should not be used for diagnosing or treating a health problem or disease. It is not a substitute for professional care. If you have or suspect you may have a health problem, you should consult your health care provider.

Table of Contents

How it started

When I was young, I developed an incredibly wide range of allergies. This made enjoying common foods like citrus, sunflower, strawberries, red apples, and chocolate impossible. From one year to the next, the list of food to stay away from grew to at least 30 other items, significantly narrowing down my choices. I also developed severe allergies to pollen, plants, pets, and dust. In total, I had about 70 or more allergies.

My first real memory of having allergies was when I was four years old. My parents and older sister were sitting in the kitchen around the table, eating fresh oranges. The memory is still very vivid. I watched them eat oranges: I smelled the delicious fruit, and saliva filled my mouth. I wanted an orange too, and asked for one. But my parents told me that I couldn't have it, because I would die from the allergic reaction. Of course, this didn't mean that my family had to stop enjoying oranges altogether just because of me. In the end, their perception was that "life is tough," and I had to learn how to deal with my limitations—and how to go without. Since that time, I remember hundreds of situations when my family enjoyed something I couldn't have. Eventually, I learned to live with it.

My parents are both doctors: they believed that I was born with allergies, and that they could not be cured. Their diagnosis was that I had an unsolveable, genetic link to an autoimmune disease. At four years old, I had to learn how to live with using medications almost every day. My parents didn't know what they didn't know: their medical training taught them that incurable diseases exist. (They were wrong: **all diseases can be cured**.) The difference is that not all **people** can be cured, such as those who would follow the advice of a doctor (like my parents) and still get sicker and sicker each year.

To make a long story short, by the beginning of the third decade of my life, I had hit rock bottom. I calculated that by that time I had consumed at least 6,000 pills to relieve my allergies. I was also exposed to all sorts of medications, as my parents were diligently following the rules of modern medicine and were giving me all sorts of concoctions for every ailment I had. They had the answer to everything in a form of a pill: red, pink, blue—you name it—they had it. It was forced upon me whether I wanted it or not.

When I hit the rock bottom, I was very sick most of the time. I had to lie in bed for weeks (especially if it was spring—the dreaded allergies season). My blood pressure would rise up out of control: 150/100. I would see stars in my eyes, I would feel dizzy, and I would always be sick. I would have allergy hives that would not go away. My face would swell to uncomfortable proportions, and my eyes would itch so bad that, at times, I considered scratching my eyes out. I would rub my eyes so much—and so hard—that I would literally rub all of my eyelashes out. I would break out so badly that the doctors would start giving me steroids to "fix" the problem.

I felt suffocated, scared, and threatened by the trees and plants during spring. I was nicknamed "a girl in a bubble" because I couldn't do anything outdoors. I couldn't even go out to dinner with friends, because any ingredient I was allergic to in the restaurant would send me straight to the hospital. My body was giving up on me, as if whole my immune system had completely crashed. Even worse, if something didn't change—and soon— it felt like the only relief would come when I stopped breathing entirely.

There was no way out with traditional doctors and medicine! At that time, I had a long-time friend who was Native American. He had a great influence on my life and he himself lived by the laws of nature. His entire family looked at doctors as people that simply cannot be trusted (and even as killers, in some cases). While he and his family may represent an extreme viewpoint, my friend is an extraordinary example of a person that has never taken a pill—not even an aspirin. His mother taught him the secrets of healthy living from childhood. He has always consumed organic foods and stays away from processed foods.

He told me that he would help me "fix" my health problems, and that all my allergies would be gone. I remember falling asleep laughing to myself, thinking: "Come on, allergies are a genetic disorder; you can't cure it. My parents know better, they are doctors! You can't cure my limitations, I'm just a sick person—that's all." But he began leading me into another reality; a reality of possibilities, where you can be cured from anything, and where simplicity is the answer. By "cured," I mean that you can create a beneficial situation for your body, where you are enabling and empowering it to fix itself—it just needs the right environment. If you want to expedite the process, you can even help your body detox toxic matter that is hard to come out on its own. I was surprised to learn that it was just a matter of time, discipline, and persistence to regain my health.

After this long journey, I dramatically improved from my limitations, both from allergies and other physical ailments. I had a bad knee since the age of six, and it got progressively worse over time. In my 20s, my knee went completely out a couple of times, and I would have to walk on crutches for six months at a time. I am now cured from arthritis on my knee. I also had a bad liver since the age of four, and that condition brought even more limitations to my diet (as well as more pills that were given to me by my parents). In addition to that, I had a herniated disk: for about a decade, it was very hard to be active. I don't have limitations any longer. That's why I decided to share with you this wonderful journey. Don't get me wrong, it was very difficult. At times, I thought it was impossible—but it was incredibly rewarding!

I will talk about toxicity in detail in this book, but if I were to tell you in one paragraph: I was getting rid of toxicity, and I was sick until most of the toxins left my system. Moreover, once I cleaned up my diet, I initially got much sicker—once you stop putting poisons inside of you, your body finally gets a chance to "unload" all the stored toxins that you accumulated over the decades. That means that your body will start melting away those stored toxins and "spit" them in your blood stream. You get high amounts of toxins in your blood stream, and you start feeling really sick until the toxins leave your body through your blood stream and exit through your lungs, skin, urine, and excrement. This process might take weeks, months, or even years.

This is a basic predominant misconception that people carry: they think if they cleaned up their diet, they should feel great right away. When they suddenly start feeling sick (which is simply one of the symptoms of detoxing), they assume that the "new" diet didn't work for them and they get back to the usual habits of what they were doing before. Once they revert to their old ways and eat toxic foods, the body switches from "unloading" old toxins to trying to cope with new, incoming ones. As your body starts storing toxins again, you might feel okay and even great for the short term—but this will result in disaster in the long run. Storing toxins is an accumulative process, meaning it takes time to store up enough toxins before that buildup is expressed in some kind of physical sickness. It could be five years down the road, or it could be 30—the timing may be different, but everyone can expect negative results.

The release of toxins can be a dangerous cycle to maneuver. If you were to take a blood test in the first week of a clean diet and then, a year later, take another blood test (while on the same diet), your blood will show a much higher level of toxins a year later. This is because your body is now releasing toxins instead of storing them. It's a very rocky road, and if you are not careful, you might drown in your own toxins. I almost did, because I wanted to get over it fast; I pushed hard, until I nearly died by drowning my system in my own toxins. My body couldn't cope with the tremendous amounts of toxins I was releasing. My parents, being good doctors, tried to convince me that my raw food lifestyle was killing me, and that you can't survive on "two pieces of lettuce" a day (as they referred to my diet). They insisted that I start eating meat and bread immediately. Only then would I feel better and heal. It was hard to go against my parents and the old beliefs that they instilled in me: after all, they are the "real" doctors, and they "know better."

David Wolfe, the famous raw foodist that has been living a raw lifestyle for decades, said: "If you want to look like a person you are taking advice from, and want to be like them (health-wise), then do exactly what they do and take their advice to heart by all means." There was no question that I admire and love my parents dearly—but did I want to be like them, health-wise? My mother had issues with rheumatoid arthritis for decades. She had high blood pressure and was always taking pills. She didn't feel well a lot of times (though she always pushed through it). She would get a cold and/or flu at least five times a year. My mom developed extreme allergies in older ages that turned into asthma, and she used an inhaler in addition to pills. My dad has always had issues with blood pressure. He has diabetes. He constantly battles with an inflamed prostate (with suspicion of developing cancer). He also grows all sorts of tumors that he cuts out of his body periodically. He always has extremely black circles under his eyes (a sign of his liver not working properly, though some people still think it's about not having enough rest). And he went bald really fast: he already had problems with hair loss in his 40s.

I definitely didn't want to be like either of my parents, health-wise. I started digging, researching. With the help and tremendous support of my Native American friend, I discovered the truth about how to regain health. A few years of persistent attention to changes in habits can lead to good health, youth, and well-being. It can completely erase worries about being sick (or running up insurmountable medical bills from hospital visits, doctors, and dependencies on pills and other treatments). And because your body is no longer deteriorating rapidly, the aging process will slow down, too. After all, aging is a sign of toxicity. Aging is not defined by the number of years. It's defined by how much toxins are accumulated in your body over decades of using it as a trash can.

With so many real, life-changing benefits, those few years dedicated to changing habits were more than worth it—they were life-saving.

Set of beliefs and our society

Food is a very sensitive subject. Everyone has his/her own opinion about foods and the best, most beneficial diet. Our whole society and customs are built around food. When you meet with your friends, you sit around the table and eat while socializing. For example, it is typical of Russian culture to greet the guest and offer food when they come to your house. If the guests refuse to join for dinner, it might be taken as an insult. Celebrating a birthday in nearly every culture includes food and cake. If you visit your family, it's about your favorite comfort foods. If there is a party, there will most likely be processed foods. No matter where you go—to the mall, the movies—food is everywhere.

Food is also in our thought processes. We spend a lot of time each day wondering what to eat for lunch or dinner. We plan and fantasize about our next sushi roll or slice of pizza. Sometimes we can't wait to leave work to go home and stuff ourselves. We **reward** ourselves with food, because that's how we are raised. Do you remember this from your childhood? "If you are a good boy/girl," or "If you do this and that, I will buy you ice cream, cookies, or your favorite treat?" That sense of reward associated with food as a child doesn't just disappear in adulthood.

And we never question what is it that we are really putting in our bodies, or how our bodies cope with all of that. We never know (or ever ask) where that meal comes from, and what type of processing it went through, or which kind of chemicals and neurotoxins were added to it. It may sound harsh, but it's true: we treat our body like a garbage can.

Another established social belief is that if you don't eat, you will die. Sick people in the hospitals get fed regardless of whether they want to or not. They are fed their "protein," for example, in the form of chicken soup so they can "get better." Let me ask you: have you ever seen a sick animal in nature that would force itself to eat when it's sick to get enough protein? The answer is NO. When the animal feels sick, it stops eating so it can heal faster (in other words, the animal is fasting). Have you ever seen a person die from starvation? There are people dying left and right from toxicity (i.e., they drown in their own toxins), but people who are skinny and look anorexic are believed to be dying due to not eating. People that die from "starvation" in third-world countries don't have clean water. They ingest all sorts of parasites, bacteria, and fungus with the dirty water, which is more likely to be blamed for their deaths than "starvation."

In addition, if a normal person breaks a water fast (as in "starvation") with the food that those starving people eat, even a normal person might die. You can't break the fast with processed, canned food that is full of toxins and think it will help. People that "die from starvation" lead this type of lifestyle: intermittent fasting with dirty water—well, in other words, starvation, while in between those "intermittent fasts," they ingest whatever they can find, and in most of the cases it's the food that should not even be suitable for human consumption.

When someone is fasting (water fasting, or dry-fasting), they have to follow the rules of how to lead in and lead out of their fasting. Otherwise, it might lead to a tragic outcome. Instead of healing themselves with fasting, they can actually hurt themselves. For example, if I didn't eat for 15 days and barely had any water, then loaded on canned food or beef and steak, fries, and beer, I just might end up in the hospital—that is, if I were lucky enough not to go into coma and die.

I want to bring up one famous case of a lady who was dry fasting for seven days (no food, no water). On the eighth day, she was supposed to lead out with water followed by extremely diluted juices (specifically avoiding citrus for the following week). Well, she decided to drink a gallon of straight orange juice instead. As a result, she was in a coma within an hour and she died the following day. Did she die from starvation? No. If you don't lead out of your fast properly, you will put your body into severe danger, which is exactly what happened to her.

Let's get back to those people that die from "starvation" in third-world countries. We can safely assume that they eat random foods that are donated. They might go without any food at all for days. If some random food is given to them—they will eat it, no matter what it is. In some really poor neighborhoods, residents will literally bake dirt and eat it to fill their stomachs. Dirt is full of all sorts of parasites, bacteria, and toxic matter that is not suitable for human consumption. Starving people also go for a number of days drinking only dirty water (and nothing else).

Is their state of "starvation" awfully similar to fasting? If so, they don't lead out of their fasting the proper way, which very likely would lead to health issues and possibly death. Let me ask you: do they die from not eating? Or do they die from not eating the right foods when breaking their involuntary fast? Do they consume clean water while they are "fasting"? If your health is already compromised and you eat—but you eat the wrong foods that are very toxic for you—will it have a severe affect on your body? I personally have never seen any person die from starvation, and until I see one with my own eyes, I will never believe such a thing exists.

I hear a lot of deaths from starvation propaganda on news feeds, which is not scientifically supported. I believe that there is a lot of "fear porn" out there with propaganda that we all have to eat (and eat a lot) to be well. Someone's got to consume all that "food" that they mass produce and push on people. At the same token, let's say they are right and you have to eat (the more the better) in order to "be healthy." This results in a very unique dilemma; by this assumption, people that eat the most should be the healthiest. But the exact opposite is true: people that are obese and eat the most are the **least** healthy. Lab testing on rats concluded that if rats are underfed, their lives are actually extended, compared to rats that are eating in abundance.

A good example of not dying from not eating would be Hira Ratan Manek (HRM)—he is an Indian man, and he is over 70 years old. While under 24/7 observation by a medical team, he proved, more than once, that it's possible to live on just clean water. One of his longest experiments lasted 411 days living only on water. According to LightDocumentary.com, he didn't lose much weight during that time. He still had a belly at the end of the experiment. You definitely wouldn't call him anorexic. All his tests, including blood tests, showed no deficiency of any kind. Moreover, his testosterone levels depicted that of a 28-year-old-man. Officially, Hira Ratan Manek is 28 years old on the inside, and 72 on the outside. He is in perfect health, and has superhuman abilities of not getting tired, not needing to sleep, etc. That is because all the energy that we spend to fight the toxins we put in our system every day, is available to him freely.

I can provide you with a list of people that have done something similar, but I believe it would be another conversation: about cleansing your body to the state of purity where your body can perfectly function without food. This state of super-optimal health requires too much work and too many sacrifices on physical and emotional levels; neverthless, it exists. This state of being and existence probably will not be interesting to most of the population. That would be a conversation of complete detoxing and stepping into breatharianism. I will explore this subject in my later works.

Another downfall of our society is believing in medications. The medical school system teaches future doctors how to suppress the symptoms, but never teach them how to cure the problem. It is a worldwide system, and we were trained to believe in it from generation to generation. Medications only make the matter worse in the long run, until we are accumulating so many inorganic poisonous chemicals in our bodies that we end up with cancer or something equally deadly. It requires accumulative effects that would build up over years (like 5, 10, 20, or 30 years) to end up with such a serious condition. Nowadays, it seems that processed and chemical-laden foods are so dominant that even teens and young kids are coming down with cancer.

I used to believe in doctors. Both of my parents are doctors. I used to travel with a box full of different medications, "just in case." But doctors are trained to cure symptoms, and they simply don't know better. They don't know how to cure the disease itself for good. Doctors don't take nutritional classes (shockingly, in the US, doctors are only required to take one day of nutritionnal classes). The average life span of a doctor is 70 years (if that), among which the last 20–30 years of their lives are usually a battle with all sorts of disorders, sores, pains, and diseases that start creeping up in their mid to late 30s. If they knew the secrets of staying healthy, they would be the first ones to become immortal—or at least not age rapidly, maintain all their hair, stay fit and thin, and be completely disease-free. And yet, if the true secrets to long-lasting health were out, they would be the first ones to be out of a job.

Allergy statistics have become an epidemic of their own, quadrupling over the past 10 years. Young children and teenagers are fighting cancer (which was unheard of before). If there was only one autistic child out of 1,000 kids 20 years ago, now there is one in every 100 due to heavy metal toxicity. Children that are born to severely toxic parents end up paying a high price. There are so many kids that have serious disorders at an early age, before they even learn how to walk. Yet, for most of society, it's a mystery how something like this has happened to their children.

Overall, social rules dictate how we live and what is supposed to be "healthy." A lot of beliefs are handed down from generation to generation without even questioning what, how, and why. The blooming of the corporate businesses pushes food producers to worry about high production—never high quality. Pesticides, toxic preservatives, and emulsifiers creep into our foods more and more. Monsanto is pushing GMO products all over the world. I've heard some producers even manage to inject organic watermelons with hormones so that they ripen faster. Watermelons are not tested for this hormone, which makes it possible to get away with producing poisonous watermelons.

Our doctors are brainwashed for eight to 10 years at schools for giving "the right pill" to people, and they don't know any better. People put their lives in the hands of those doctors without question. It's time to take matters into your own hands by researching, finding out the truth, and taking full responsibility for your own health. No more excuses. I am not encouraging you to fight the system, nor to try to convince others. In the end we do need doctors, such as in cases when someone gets in a car accident and is brought to the hospital in pieces. Only doctors can stitch them together and save his/her life. All I encourage is this: if you feel like the information in this book resonates with you—if traditional medicine has offered no cure—and you want to improve your health, then this book can help raise the questions for you to research and test the findings on your own system in order to get to the bottom of the real truth.

Are people really fat?

The majority of population is obese in the US. It's an epidemic that has taken over the best of everyone, including children. It's very rare when you see a child and he/she's not overweight. I used to think that it works like this; let's say you eat 2,000 calories a day. If you use/burn the same 2,000 calories a day, you are not going to be fat. If you only use half of what you eat, that's when you will get fat. That's the basic idea that they taught me at the University of Minnesota when I took nutrition classes. Extra weight is just extra, unused energy that is turned into fat and stored away in your body.

I don't believe that anymore. According to my research, it's much simpler. You consume food that is toxic and your body is trying to cope with toxins. So, it tries to retain and store more water in each cell to dilute all that garbage (toxins). With time, the toxins get accumulated more and more. The liver is overloaded and can barely function; it can't cope with all the toxins, so the body stores it anywhere it can in an effort to save itself. Your body stores toxins in the gallbladder by forming stones (to entrap and encapsulate the toxins); in joints; in tissue; and in muscles. Once all that toxic matter is stored away, the body needs to dilute those toxins and get even more water into the cells so the cells can function and not drown in all that toxic waste. To put it plainly, this is exactly how people get fat.

For example, if you eat organic clean carrots, you can eat 20 pounds a day, and won't gain weight (in many cases in the US, you most likely will lose weight). This is because it doesn't have all the toxins that wheat bread or processed food has. If you eat bread instead of carrots—that's a different story. Your body has a hard time coping with such huge levels of toxins (like any processed foods would have), and it has to retain more and more water to deal with it.

I will go deeper into the details about each type of toxic foods and why they are so

The results showed that women that drank milk developed osteoporosis and brittle bones. But women that didn't drink milk were healthy. This research was working against the corporation, so they suppressed the results of the study to push their agenda on people to make big bucks. In this example, we can see that the toxins in milk leached calcium from the bones of those women. Those women accumulated more toxins and mucus in their systems (and I will get into the harsh reality of toxicity of dairy products later on). Your body can create a perfect balance on its own and it doesn't require much at all once it rids of all the chemicals, heavy metals, and toxins you put in it.

As another example, if you have heavy metal toxicity, those heavy metals block the absorption of minerals and vitamins resulting in deficiencies. Lead is a heavy metal and is toxic to our system. If you have lead in your system, then it will pretend to act as calcium. Therefore, your body will not absorb calcium, because those receptors are already taken and blocking the absorption of real calcium. The best comparison would be if the receptor is a bottle, lead is a cork in that bottle. Calcium can't be used unless we get rid of the lead first. What happens is that your body is malfunctioning and you develop deficiencies. And even if you put a huge amount of calcium in your body, it will exit without any effect. All the receptors where calcium belongs are already taken by lead.

It's not as important what you put in your system—it's what you DON'T put in your system that matters. For example, people are looking for that "magic pill" that will cure it all. If they see some new vitamins or superfoods, and some magic mushroom powders, they think that they will find the answer—but this is not the case. Like I said, it's not what you are putting in your system, it's what you are **not** putting in it. If you are eating raw fruits, greens, and veggies, you are choosing NOT to eat fries and steak—which is an amazing gift to give your body.

If you avoid putting junk in your system, your body will self-correct over time. You do not need a magic pill, vitamin, mineral, or any other superfoods and supplements (though they might be helpful at times). It's very simple: just avoid certain foods that are very toxic for your system. If you don't do that, your body will accumulate toxins with time, and you will come down with a disastrous disorder or sickness one day. It's like sitting on a time bomb that is ticking 10 years, 20 years, 30 years...and boom! For each their own, whether it's high blood pressure, allergies, cancer, arthritis, or something else, it will show up and progress when given enough time.

It reminds me of an experiment my mother was telling me about; if you take a frog and put it in boiling water, it will start trying to jump out of it, and fight for its life. On the other hand, if you put the frog in cold water and slowly warm it up to boil, the frog will stay in the water and boil to death. Basically, it won't notice what is happening until it's too late, and that will kill it. It seems to me that we are like those frogs that are sitting in cold water: by adding more toxins each year, we don't notice how we are incrementally destroying ourselves. The accumulative process of toxins is very slow and takes decades to fully affect and destroy our body. (It's also worth mentioning that "starting to fall apart" in mid-age seems absolutely normal and expected.)

People say, "Oh, come on, you can have a bite, it won't kill you"—and they are right. You can have a bite of pizza, steak, cheese, bread, cake, and it won't kill you. At least, not right away. If it doesn't kill us right away, we think we got away with it. Unfortunately, we are wrong. We will pay the price, it's just a matter of how long it takes before that bill arrives. It does kill you, but it's not a "hard kill." It won't kill you instantly like a bullet; instead, it will be more like a "soft kill." It will take a duration of a decade or two until it catches up with you and hits you hard. It will also bring a lot of health issues and suffering when it starts to finally show a physical expression in your body. When it rains, it pours.

What does cooked food do to you?

Not many people question this one. And even less people look for an answer. Despite knowing the answer, we are too addicted to some of these foods to stop eating them—even though we know they are literally killing us. It's like a cigarette smoker: it's written on the box that it might cause cancer and other health issues, but the addict goes for another one knowing the consequences, and knowing that it's only a matter of time.

We are what we eat, no doubt about it. I highly recommend watching the documentary *Food Matters*. In this film, it was stated (based upon experiment) that cooked food is seen by the body to be toxic and that the body deploys a white cell reaction. It was further found that if at least 51% of a meal was raw, the body would have much lesser negative reaction to food and thus would not strain our already overworked immune systems.

This has to do with the food enzymes being destroyed during the cooking process.

Cooked foods act like a toxin. A raw food diet eliminates toxic response from the body. The study found that your body reacts the same way to eating cooked foods as it does when it gets infected or when it's exposed to a toxin. Once you start to eat cooked foods, white blood cells are produced in large quantities.

In 1930, a research team led by Dr. Paul Kouchakoff set out to test and document the effect of food on the immune system. Their testing (conducted at the Institute of Clinical Chemistry in Zurich, Switzerland) focused on comparing the effects of consuming cooked and processed foods versus raw and natural foods. They found that white blood cell (leukocytes) production increased immediately after eating cooked foods. Scientists call this "digestive leukocytosis," which occurs after eating cooked and processed foods, and has always been considered a normal physiological response. It was unclear as to why white blood cell production would immediately increase after eating a meal, as if the body were fighting off an infection, toxin, or responding to trauma.

The same study yielded a fascinating discovery: while cooked foods stimulated a white blood cell response, raw food did not. Highly altered food also increased white blood cells (i.e., foods with added chemicals, preservatives, sugar, etc.). Instead of referring to food-generated white blood cell production as "digestive leukocytosis," the research team renamed the process to "pathological leukocytosis."

Even the specific cooking temperature of food yielded a different white blood cell response. Foods that were cooked at too high of a temperature created a protective response, as if the body was protecting the bloodstream. But by and large, the foods that sparked the most significant white blood cell reactions (no matter whether they were cooked or not) were refined, pasteurized, homogenized, or preserved.

Francis M. Pottenger, Jr., M.D. is best known for his ten-year, multi-generational nutritional study. He studied nutritional effects on cats from 1932–1942, culminating in his book titled *Pottenger's Cats: A Study in Nutrition*. Pottenger's cat experiments have been called by DoctorYourself.com "a decade-long scientifically controlled *Supersize Me* experiment" (reference to a must-see documentary about cooked fast food affecting the human body). Basically, there were two groups of cats. The first group comprised of cats who ate the daily cat equivalent of fast food (i.e., nothing but cooked food). Another group was fed nothing but raw food. The result was not surprising: the cats that were fed raw food were thriving, and the cats that were fed cooked food were anything but. The cooked diet caused cats to develop degenerative diseases and other pathologies, none of which were observed in the cats that ate a raw diet. It's hard not to make a correlation between cooked food and diseases—and in fact, within the raw food movement, Dr. Pottenger's study has become an invaluable reference, proving that cooking food is much more dangerous than we realize.

My father (remember, he is a "real" doctor, a Ph.D. that finished the traditional medical school where he got very misinformed and brainwashed) always told me, "You can eat everything in moderation as far as our bodies are designed to fight and expel toxins. That's what our bodies do." Well, he is right that our bodies have the ability to fight the toxins— provided they are 100% functional and not compromised, and provided that we don't literally drown our system with overloads of toxic inorganic matter. My father also says that a little bit of toxins won't hurt our systems.

My question is: how much is "little" and how much is to be considered a system overload? I mean, how does this sound to you: if you drink a little bit of gasoline every day, it's OK—your body will manage as long as it's in moderation. We put toxins and neurotoxins in our systems that are much harsher than gasoline. We do it three times a day and then wonder why we have all sorts of diseases.

Another immune system response to cooked food is mucus. When cooked food is eaten, our bodies try to protect us from this invasion by creating mucus. This mucus makes a wall between the food and our bodies. Being a raw foodist for a while, if I eat any cooked food, I would be literally knocked off my feet within the first 15 minutes of ingesting the cooked food. I would feel like someone sedated or heavily drugged me, and as if someone fogged my mind. I would feel like I can't move any more. I also might feel as if I got poisoned and could start showing symptoms of food poisoning. This feeling would take couple of days to completely clear out as soon as I get back to 100% raw foods. Ingesting cooked foods requires much longer sleep time for the body to detox your system overnight. These are the real effects of cooked foods on the body of a person that has detoxed quite a bit.

The best comparison would be of an alcoholic: if the person drinks a lot of alcohol, he conditions his body to this substance and the body becomes more tolerant of alcohol (of course, at the expense of their health and deterioration of their liver). This person would be able to drink a bottle of vodka and be fine. In other words, the person won't feel very strong effects of alcohol due to constant conditioning of their body. The longer the person drinks, the more tolerance they develop. On the other hand, if the person is not used to this toxic substance, then one drink might be too much for the healthy person's liver to handle. The body will react to it immediately and notify the body that this toxic matter is in the system. This person will be under quite an influence of alcohol, with strong and unpleasant hangover symptoms afterwards.

When food is heated, the enzymes are also destroyed. Enzymes are the life force in food, the magic elixir of life. They merge with our bodies and tell us how and where to use the food we eat. It's the enzymes that tell the vitamin C in the orange to go and become part of our skin. Some believe that enzymes are destroyed by stomach acids, but research shows that enzymes are mainly absorbed in the mouth before our food gets into the stomach. Our body can't communicate with the food unless the enzymes are there. Raw food contains its own digestive enzymes and literally digests itself inside you. Raw food breaks itself down and goes where it is needed. Without its enzymes, cooked food sits in your gut like a brick and rots. Your body has to produce and use its own digestive enzymes to deal with the cooked food. Many now believe that humans only have enough digestive enzymes to last them into their 40s, if they are lucky. When enzymes are depleted, everything seems to be working harder physically, and many become apathetic and lose their zest for life.

As David Wolfe mentions, there are systemic enzymes and there are digestive enzymes. Digestive enzymes might also be systemic enzymes depending on when you use them. For example, the enzyme bromelain (derived from pineapple) could be taken with food to help with digestion, as it will play a role of a digestive enzyme. But if you take bromelain between meals, it will pass your stomach untouched, and enter your system to clean it up from unbroken matter and some toxic proteins that are accumulated in your system.

When I started my detox and went raw, I started taking "Beauty Enzymes," created by David Wolfe. It seems they are the best enzymes on the market (both systemic and digestive) that are made of plant-based matter, and provide great assistance in assimilation and absorption of foods as well as cleaning up the system.

Cooked foods are dead foods that paralyze your digestive system, overloading your body with toxins from fermentation and rot. Your body can't bear to deal with this overload that causes constipation, indigestion, and all sorts of ailments. I can totally imagine going 90 days on only raw, fresh juices, or fruits and greens without any problem. In fact, I have done it! But I can't imagine eating only cooked foods for 90 days. I tried this challenge. I ate fried potatoes for dinner (I will be honest,

I enjoyed eating them), but I felt horrible afterwards for hours (my body absolutely didn't like that). Yet, the following morning I ate more cooked roots. That was the last time I had to eat cooked foods.

I had to stop that challenge. I was getting too sick and lethargic. When you start to feel the benefits of what raw foods can do for you and how much energy you have, it's impossible to get back to that sluggish, heavy state that cooked foods bring you. The thing is, we are all conditioned to eating cooked foods. We simply don't know how it might feel on raw foods (especially after you pass the stage of the uncomfortable part of detoxing). But once you get a glimpse of how it might be, it is then that you realize the whole meaning of "being healthy." This definition is far from the traditional understanding of what we learn from society, family, and doctors.

Food addiction or lack of

discipline

Unfortunately, we are all victims of misleading conditioning, false information, and addiction to foods. For example, wheat products and dairy products contain opioid peptides. Opioid peptides are amino acids that mimic the effect of opiates in the brain. An opiate is a drug, hormone, or other chemical substance having sedative or narcotic effects similar to those containing the very addictive opium or its derivatives. Opioid peptides may be produced by the body itself, like endorphins, or be absorbed from partially digested food. The effects of these peptides vary, but they all resemble opiates.

Brain opioid peptide systems have been found to play important roles in a number of daily processes, such as food intake control, stress and pain responses, attachment behavior, emotions, and even motivation. These opioid peptides (and almost all beta-carbolines) are physically addictive, making you eat more. Think about how you feel when you pass by a bakery and get a whiff of freshly baked bread: you immediately sense yourself getting "hungry," right? This is not just because you are addicted, but also because your body has started to secrete digestion juices as soon as you caught that stimulating odor.

A raw food diet is a way to side-step the toxic and manipulative effects of all this. It's simultaneously a good thing and a bad thing. Who doesn't want to feel a sense of well-being after eating a cooked meal (after all, there is a reason they are called comfort foods)? Even if it's a false sense of well-being, it's there. You can't get this feeling from eating raw foods.

Food manufacturers are aware of the physically addictive qualities of opioid peptides and beta-carbolines. They apply this knowledge to increase and maintain the number of their customers, and to successfully compete with other food manufacturers. They know that wheat and milk protein contain the most opioid peptides, and that is why these proteins are most often added to prepared food products. They know that beta-carbolines also increase your appetite. That is why they are also added to most food products, including sauces and spices, and in so-called "taste enhancers."

How many times have you continued to eat something you didn't really like? You took a bite, and for some reason, you couldn't leave it alone until you had finished the whole package. That package of cookies might have been laying in your kitchen cabinet for a few days, but once it was opened and you had taken one bite, it kept pulling you back to get more.

Have you ever experienced this with fruit? No, you have never had to have another banana, apple, orange, or cucumber (which is a fruit) once you are full. You might love to eat fruit when you are hungry, but it never keeps pulling you back to eat some more until you finish all of them that are in your house. Now you know—you do not keep on eating because you are weak or pathetic, but because you are physically addicted to beta-carbolines and opioid peptides. If your overeating was due to some psychological reason, any food that tastes good, including ripe fruits, would be equally satisfying. But this is not the case. All of us are physically addicted to these beta-carbolines and opioid peptides.

Still, each of us is different and is susceptible to these chemicals in a different way. That's why different people prefer a different poison for themselves, such as different brands of cigarettes, alcohol, or coffee. That is why food manufacturers experiment. They add a bit more wheat protein to their products, some malt, or a bit less milk protein, or combine these with concentrates of a particular dehydrated protein heated in combination with sugar. Then, they must make sure that we are familiarized with "the taste" (their specific combination of addictive chemicals) of this new product. They strategically position their dealers in the supermarket to offer the customers a free sample. We behave according to the expectations of the food manufacturers, so we take what he/she offers us and try it. If this specific blend of addictive chemicals matches our own addiction, our brain says, "I Like It!" and the journey of starting to buy that product begins.

This strategy is the same as that applied by the "pusher" who gives drugs for free to youngsters to get them addicted and thus gains new "junkie" clients. There is essentially no fundamental difference between a drug junkie and food junkie. They both are addicted to physically addictive chemicals. They both need their fix every few hours. They just look different: the drug junkie gets skinnier and doesn't take care of his/her appearance. The food junkie becomes either overweight, obese, or moderately above the normal weight (but with health issues). Both become dependent and need larger doses of their "drug" to achieve the same effect. From my prerspective, any type of food that affects and/or manipulates the state of human being in any shape or form is considered to be a drug. That would probably be a fair 99% of all foods that humans consume on daily basis.

What are mucus-forming and mucusless foods?

I would highly recommend you read the book by Arnold Ehret titled *Mucusless Diet Healing System*. Arnold was very sick and literally dying by the age of 30. After spending thousands of dollars on doctors and getting even worse after their treatments, he was at a dead end. Doctors were helpless and gave up on him. He had to go on his own search to win his health back. He experimented a lot on his own body with foods, and he completely healed himself through proper eating and fasting.

In his book, he explains that foods could be mucus-forming and mucusless. The mucus-forming foods are destructive to our health. They stick to the walls of intestines, layer upon layer, forming a mucoid plaque that poisons your system and prevents absorption of nutrients. Within the decades of build-up, the plaque might reach the thickness of over one inch and narrow down the passage in your intestines.

Mucus-forming foods would be all dairy products, breads, all processed and cooked foods, and most grains. Quinoa and buckwheat are much less mucus-forming and, therefore, healthier choices. (They are both technically seeds, not grains.) He encourages you to conduct your own experiment—for example, to take rice and boil it. Then, strain water from it and you will see paste or a glue-like liquid (actually, you can glue things with it). And that's exactly what is happening inside of you. If you consume mucus-forming foods, your intestines get glued-up, layer upon layer all over the intestinal walls, and food gets stuck and rots inside of you till it turns into fecal stones that are stuck to your intestinal walls. This hardened fecal matter blocks the absorption of nutrients and turns all that buildup into toxic matter.

On the other hand, Arnold suggests you take grapes (or juiced grapes) and boil them. No matter how long you boil them, it will not turn into glue. The grape substance will get thicker if you evaporate water, but you won't be able to glue anything with it, and that would define this type of food as mucusless.

Arnold suggests fruits and raw foods to melt away all that thick fecal matter that encrusts your intestinal walls. In his book, he gives specifics of what would work best and what won't. He also published pictures of himself when he was sick in his 30s (and he looked like an old man), and then pictures in his 50s (when he got completely detoxed, healthy, and radiant—and he looked 30 in his 50s).

The general rule is: dairy, breads, flour, grains, meats, and animal products are all mucus-forming foods. All fruits and veggies are not mucus-forming. There are exceptions to this rule: for example, starchy veggies like potatoes, are mucus-forming.

I am a true believer that it is best to take advice from someone that proved on their own body that their idea works (in his case, Arnold actually cured hundreds of patients with the help of his diet, including himself). At the age of 50, Arnold looked 20 years younger his age. Through his research and experiments on his own body, he proved that the human body functions best on a fruitarian diet. He lived a fruitarian lifestyle for decades.

While on fruits, he intently cut his arm and it took him two days to heal with no scar left behind. Then he switched to SAD (Standard American Diet) by eating meat, potatoes, and other mucus-forming and cooked foods, chasing it with beer. After that, he intently cut his arm again. This time, after eating mucus forming, cooked, and processed foods, his cut was barely healing. It took him two weeks to get better, but he had to go back to fruits to completely heal, and only then he healed with a scar left behind. It's very curious that in our society, we know that the average recovery time after surgery is about 10 to 14 days. That's what Arnold proved on his own body after eating cooked and unhealthy foods. But imagine if you cut a person's body that is clean and detoxed. Maybe the healing time might be only two to four days.

Arnold was killed in his 50s because, I assume they didn't want people to get super healthy and live forever. All economy would fall apart if that happened. Who would be consuming all medications, undergoing all the harmful treatments, and using the services of doctors? In official records it was stated that he slipped, fell down, and died. The usual story, wouldn't you say? If not for his "accident," he probably would have lived for a very, very long time, and would have been an example of "how to make it work" in the long run. He would have been an exemplary example of perfect health with minimum effects of aging and outstanding quality of life.

In the recent years, there are a lot of holistic doctors that paid with their lives, because they went against the established system of pill feeding and widely accepted harmful treatments. For example, some people shoot themselves in the back of their head a couple of times and then go and throw themselves off the bridge. There are over 87 deaths of holistic doctors that used non-traditional medicine and actually cured the patients permanently, but ended up "committing suicide." Some of them, being stable and happy and never showing any signs of depression, suddenly become "depressed" and "take" their whole families with them. The best part is when they shoot themselves not once, but twice in the back of their own heads...go figure. I really hope I won't have to pay the same price for revealing the truth. I am not depressed, nor suicidal, but you never know when I "might decide to shoot myself in the back of my head few times, then shoot my family; yet after that, go and throw myself and my family off the bridge..." You never know nowadays...

Getting back to natural holistic healing, Johanna Brandt would take it even further. One of her patients had cancer and she helped her heal through two months of an only-grapes diet (you can learn the details in her book, *The Grape Cure*). Yet Arnold Ehret did extensive experiments on himself by water fasting for 80 days (two months) in a row. Then, he would break it with prunes and go on a three-day hiking trip with no rest (because neither him, nor another person that he did this fasting with were tired, so they didn't need to sleep for three days).

Arnold went back and forth from fasting to cooked foods just to experience the effects of those types of foods on his health. After that, he concluded that cooked foods as well as mucus-forming foods were detrimental to human health. Arnold Ehret's books were the first ones that I read on the way to infinite health when I started my journey. His books became like a Bible to me. I am really grateful for his work.

What are acidic and alkaline foods? What is pH?

When we are in an acidic state, we experience many health problems. Acidity constricts you, causing stiffness and tissue degeneration. Alkalinity does the opposite: our bodies can release tension and stress, and our blood and lymph can flow more easily. Being in an alkaline state is absolutely lovely. Alkalinity soothes away our health problems and we become balanced, calm, and peaceful.

The scale that is used for measuring the pH, or hydrogen ion concentration, is from 0 to 14, with 7 being the neutral point. Below 7 is acidic and above 7 is alkaline. The optimal pH of the body's fluids, such as the blood and urine, is 7.0 to 7.4, slightly alkaline. Outside this range, the body's activity is no longer optimal and the metabolism is out of balance.

The pH of the body is largely influenced by metabolic byproducts and by our diet. Thus, pH is directly affected by the various categories of foods that we eat and the internal mechanisms involved in their processing. Some foods that are acidic in their composition can become alkalinizing following metabolization by the body, such as lemons. Accordingly, it is important to be more aware of the impact that various foods in our diet have on the internal environment of the body.

When your system is acidic, this allows oxidation, which leads to decay. Too much acidity brings a whole host of health problems, the most noticeable of which are often weakened teeth, skin, hair, and bones. According to StepsToLife.org, additional effects of acidity that may not be so noticeable on the surface include:

- Deterioration of the digestive tract
- Leaky gut syndrome
- Candida
- Allergies
- Excitability of the nervous system
- Sciatica
- Tendency to depressive illness

- Anxiety
- Panic disorders
- Muscular spasms and cramps
- Enhanced susceptibility to infections
- Chronic fatigue
- Blockage of certain minerals which become unavailable
- Increased risk of cancerous cells proliferating

When the fluids of the human body are maintained at a healthy alkaline level (7.0 – 7.4), it protects the body from bacteria, viruses and fungi, while also bringing for the life-giving form inherent within the hydrogen matrix. Accordingly, an acidic pH breaks down the normal functioning of the biological systems, resulting in degenerative conditions within the body and providing a receptive environment for chronic inharmonies (i.e., disease).

The following factors will have an influence on the pH of the body:

1) **Acidic Foods** such as fast foods, meats, processed grains, refined salt, sugar,

condiments (pickles, ketchup, etc.), soda, and all other refined and processed foods (including commercial flours) have a pH ranging from 2.8 to 5.5, which is highly acidic. These foods tear down our health.

2) **Alkaline Foods** such as fruits, almonds, unpasteurized honey, bee pollen, figs, dates, raw earth/root vegetables, green vegetables, apricots, avocados, coconut, grapes, molasses, raisins and lemons will all restore our health.

We are at our absolute best when our bodies are alkaline. Alkaloid highs like caffeine, cocaine, or marijuana are what helps us recreate the alkaline sensation. The problem with these drugs, however, is that they leave us even more acidic when they disappear, meaning we will need more of them to return to that same aklaline feeling.

Our cultural belief is that we have to eat animal products for "protein," and we have to eat cooked foods for "nutrients." Over the decades, we become severely toxic from processed and cooked foods. In addition to this, all the chemicals that we are exposed to by using soaps, shampoos, lotions, makeup, hair dyes, frying pans, utensils, plastic storage containers, cups, and environmental pollution also increase the toxicity in our body. Toxicity is highly correlated with acidity; the more toxic you are, the more acidic you become.

Also, the pH of the body is greatly influenced by your emotions. In his book, *The Chronic Stress Crisis*, Dr. William G. Timmins says: "Joyous, happy, love-filled emotions tend to create alkaline-forming chemical reactions in the body. Conversely, emotions that are filled with anger, fear, jealousy, and hate create acid-forming chemical reactions in the body. This is done through the master gland, the hypothalamus, which is controlled by our thoughts, emotions, and attitude." This master gland (often referred to as the mind-body connection) controls the entire endocrine system (producing numerous hormones, neurotransmitters and chemicals) and the parasympathetic nervous system.

The question then arises about how to bring the pH of the "body fluids" into an acceptable range, that lies between 7.0 and 7.4, which will then influence the blood to maintain its optimal 7.4 pH level. My best choice would be juicing greens. You can add an apple for flavor, but try to juice at least a quart of green drinks a day consistently for a month, and you will see the difference. That was my ritual for months and months with no end; to start every morning with green juice until I became a 100% fruitarian and my pH was stable between 7.2 and 7.4. If I went on a business trip, I would take a juicer with me and juiced the first thing in the morning in any hotel I was staying at. I would not miss a day. My favorite juice would consist of 4–5 cups of organic spinach, half of a large head of celery, and one large apple.

Why did I chose to do it in the morning? Firstly, celery is very hydrating (at the beginning stage of transition, when you go from an all-American cooked foods diet to a vegan and raw vegan diet). Secondly, celery has all the vital salts that are needed for your proper digestion throughout the day.

Once you become a 100% fruitarian, you might find celery dehydrating because of its high salt content. You might even experience a dry mouth as if you were eating salt. But as long as you are eating mixed foods and using salt in your foods, celery juice will actually be helpful, as it would regulate your bowel movement and eliminate intestinal discomfort.

Spinach has a lot of chlorophyll, which is chemically similar to the hemoglobin found in human blood. Chlorophyll is the most powerful cleansing and purifying agent available in nature. In fact, they are so similar that they only have one key difference: in chlorophyll, the central atom is magnesium. In human blood, the central atom is iron. Chlorophyll has significant benefits as a food supplement. Not only can it help detoxify and purify your liver and your blood, but it can also aid in creating red blood cells and help with tissue repair. One of the best detoxifying superfoods that is high in chlorophyll would be wheat grass juice, and you can add it to any drink or smoothie you choose. It also has all the needed nutrients and minerals for the body's building blocks, hence wheat grass juice is called a "superfood."

While we are sleeping through the night, we are "fasting." When we wake up, we are very acidic due to the all-night detoxification that your body tries to do every night. I found it really energizing when you balance your pH in the morning by drinking juiced spinach to bring your alkalinity up after a night of detoxing. I would call my morning juice "breakfast," where I would break the night "fast" with highly alkaline juice. I usually add an apple in my juice just for the taste. Sometimes, I would add one-quarter of an inch of ginger root to my juice for the flavor and for its beneficial properties (it's anti-bacterial, anti-inflammatory, and great for your digestive system).

Wheatgrass shots are awesome as well, but if you are very toxic, you might not feel so good after drinking it—so be very careful with wheatgrass. I would not recommend drinking it more than once a day starting with a very small amount, and very slowly increasing the dose. I also read that if you drink 2–3 ounces of wheatgrass every day, it might help even with curing cancer. However, wheatgrass is considered to be a superfood, so please be respectful of this fact and remember that sometimes less is more.

Another key factor is the water that we drink. Water accounts for up to 75% of the human body weight, thus the fluidic intake greatly impacts the pH of the body. I never drank water from the sink (it has a low pH and is extremely toxic). I always preferred Reverse Osmosis water because of our environmental pollution. The pollution in big cities made me feel unsafe to ingest unfiltered water. Reverse Osmosis water is not an optimal solution, but I used what was easily available at that time.

In order to balance your pH, the easiest choice would be alkaline-forming raw and untreated foods that could be introduced into your diet on a regular basis such as apricots, cucumbers, avocados, lemons, oranges, coconuts, melons, figs, dates, grapes, other fruits, greens, sprouts, veggies, and almonds. Note: when consuming almonds, soaking them for 24 hours prior to consumption starts the germination process in the seed and thus activates its life force. As a result, the digestive system is able to assimilate more of the elements contained within the almonds. There is a long list of fruits, vegetables, and seeds that you can Google to see the entire table of foods that are highly alkaline and beneficial for you. Such foods will help you bring up your pH.

It is a good practice to be aware of the alkaline/acid condition of your body. The pH is measured by a urine or saliva test, which is very simple to do and requires less than a minute of your time. Hydrion pH Testing Strips, which are available through most drug stores and some health food stores, are the best tool for measuring your pH. These are color coded into a general pH range. You should look for test strips that will register half-point increments. When using these test strips as your guideline, try to balance the body pH between 7 and 7.4. I highly doubt that any person that eats cooked food or the (SAD) Standard American Diet would even reach the mark of 6.0. (At least, I have not met any person who doesn't have pH higher then 6.0 while eating the SAD diet.)

Also, keep in mind that the best time to take an accurate pH reading would be the first thing in the morning, when you get up before brushing your teeth or drinking or eating anything. That would be the true pH of your body. If you measure your body's pH level during the day or between meals, it will not be accurate. It will be much higher than your true pH. This is because any food and drink you have already consumed during that day will influence the pH level. Very often, I see people stating that their pH is close to 7.4, or even 8.0, yet they have all sorts of health issues. Why? Because if you just ate or drank anything, it will affect the result, especially if you ate highly alkaline foods. You should wait 4–5 hours and not eat or drink anything to measure the correct pH level. This means that the best time to measure your pH would be in the morning. Also, it will be the lowest point of your pH where you will see the true picture of where you are at. When the body is working to detox throughout the night, it will become more acidic, especially if you are toxic and have something to detox. Therefore, you will see the true depiction of your body's condition in the morning. Once you are able to achieve and sustain your pH at about 7.0–7.4 while taking the proper measurements in the mornings, only then you are truly healthy.

What happens when the body is acidic? The body will try to compensate for the acidic pH by using alkaline minerals and it will deplete minerals from your body to cope with the situation. An acidic pH of the body will decrease the body's ability to absorb minerals and other nutrients, deplete the energy production in the cells, limit its ability to repair damaged cells, decrease its ability to detoxify heavy metals, make tumor cells thrive, and make it more susceptible to fatigue and illness.

The typical American diet is exremely high in acid-producing foods (animal products such as eggs, dairy, and meat) and extremely low in alkaline-producing foods (such as fresh fruits and vegetables). And the processed foods that we eat are all acid-producing, too. White flour, sugar, coffee, and soda are all stimulating acid production in our bodies. Even artificial sweeteners can be toxic, such as NutraSweet, Sweet'N'Low, and Splenda. One of the best things we can do to correct an overly acidic body is to clean up the diet and lifestyle.

To maintain good health, your diet should include at least 60% alkaline-forming foods and 40% acid-forming foods (please keep in mind that if you eat vegetables, they are alkaline, but if you cook the same vegetables, they become acidic). To restore health, your diet should include at least 80% alkaline-forming foods and 20% acid-forming foods. Try to fill your daily diet with fresh fruits and veggies to strive for optimal health.

Are Himalayan salts safe?

One of the most frequently debated isues in the US is, without a doubt, food safety. A significant complication in the US is that the USDA and FDA often partner with manufacturers to promote food products for profit (rather than focusing on the safety and well-being of American citizens). Salt recommendations are monitored by the FDA, which includes natural salts.

According to an article written by Dr. Gayle Eversole on Rense.com: "Original Himalayan Crystal Salt Elements" lists only 84 "natural", 100% pure elements needed by the body. These include: hydrogen, lithium, beryllium, boron, carbon, nitrogen, oxygen, fluoride, sodium, magnesium, aluminum, cilium, phosphorus, sulfur, chloride, calcium, scandium, titanium, vanadium, chromium, manganese, iron, cobalt, nickel, copper, zinc, gallium, garmanium, arsenic, selenium, bromine, rubidium, strontium, yttrium, zirconium, niobium, molybdenum, ruthenium, rhodium palladium, silver, cadmium, indium, tin, antimony, tellurium, iodine, cesium, barium, lanthanum, cerium, praseodymium, samarium, europium, gadolinium, terbium, dysprosium, holmium, erbium, thulium, ytterbium, lutetium, hafnium, tantalum, tungsten, rhenium, osmium, iridium, platinum, gold, mercury, thallium, lead, bismuth, polonium, astatine, francium, radium, actinium, thorium, protactinium, uranium, neptunium and plutonium.

Interestingly enough, the company does not offer a chemical analysis report on their own product. Dr. Gayle Eversole noticed a few elements known to be toxic from her studies of chemistry and some radioactive elements, in order to make a point. Her findings led her to believe that these elements are not "needed by the body."

Her review of another supplier of Himalayan salt does provide a chemical analysis for the toxic heavy metals and fluoride. In this product, she found 192 PPM (parts per million) of fluoride. In a third product, she found 16 PPM of fluoride. According to Dr. Eversole's research, it seems as though consumers are simply not being given the information they need in order to make the best decisions for their health.

Don't forget that exposure to fluoride is cumulative. The damage won't happen right away—it occurs over time. And over the course of our lifetime, we are exposed to high levels of this toxic element through air pollution, municipal water, prescription drugs, and even the kinds of foods we ingest.

I also read another idea about "healthy salts" which I chose to believe. I read that it is OK to use Himalayan Pink salt in emergency situations (kind of like a "natural" pill) to restore the electrolyte balance in the body if the person feels sick. Despite that, it shouldn't be used on daily basis at all. When you take vitamins and minerals, they should be bio-available to you in order to be able to process them and be used by your system. So, if you push those minerals and vitamins through the plant while it's growing, they will become bio-available to you when you consume that plant. If you try to take inert minerals straight out of soil (I am not sure how many people would enjoy eating dirt), they won't be processed and dealt with by your body as they are not bio-avalilable to your system. In response, our body will try to store those elements anywhere and everywhere it can if it's already overloaded with incoming other toxins from foods you consume on daily basis. Your body reacts to salt like it's a toxin, or inorganic matter, and whatever your system can't remove, it will try to encapsulate to protect the body (provided your system can't process and get rid of it shortly after consumption, which is the case for 99.9% of population that overwhelm their bodies with toxins). It's an accumulative effect, and five, 10, or may be 15 years down the road, suddenly you might feel pain in your joints and develop arthritis, or have other health issues, or some other inflammatory disease as a result of the stored-up toxins.

Salt is a very strong stimulant. Anyone can understand the meaning of the word "stimulant," but not everyone can actually realize what it really means. Let me tell you about my experience, where I felt as if I had six cups of coffee at once. It happened after a long time of abstinence from salt in my diet. One day, shortly after consumption of salted foods, my blood pressure shot out of control; I felt a throbbing pounding in my head that soon turned into a migraine. I felt like I had to drink gallons and gallons of water to quench my thirst, and to bring my body back in balance. My mouth was burning from the inside (like the salt had eroded everything in my mouth). That convinced me that we are meant to live without salt.

Please don't take my word for it, as my opinions are based on my experiences and results of my own research. I encourage you to go though your own experiences, and put the knowledge in this book to test. I suggest that you go salt-free for three weeks, and then eat it again with your meals. I want you to see how your body would react to the first meal with salt. If you don't try it, you will always be in doubt of why salt is called a stimulant, and to what extent it affects a person. Have you ever questioned why we don't feed salt to infants? Why all baby food doesn't have salt? Only after months and months of conditioning the infant with small doses of salt, we can then start feeding him/her that toxic substance in their meals. As a matter of fact, if you give a newborn a pickle, the infant will be in great discomfort and most likely would have diarrhea and a stomachache. However, as adults, we have the strangest assumption that we NEED salt in our diet and we have to add table salt to all our foods.

It's actually interesting to mention that after extensive fasting, when I started eating a tomato, I realized that it was so darn salty on its own. I never knew the real taste of this fruit, because I used all sorts of dressings on my salads and tomatoes (or I would put a dash of salt on it). By using condiments for the duration of our entire lives, we desensitize our taste buds, and live in the world of "warped" perceptions because of it. If you clean up your diet, you will heighten your senses and realize how colorful the taste of plain fruits and vegetables are. You will have to re-introduce the whole world of tasting to yourself.

Once, after five days of dry fasting (I will discuss this type of fasting further in this book), the second week after I came out of it, I tried to put a little bit of salt on cucumber and developed a severe migraine right after eating it. I couldn't believe that such a tiny amount of salt would send me to "hell" for hours until the next day. So, I tried to use salt for a few more days in a row, and each time I would end up with a migraine. It took me two weeks to condition myself to being able to use a little bit of salt without developing a severe migraine, but I would still get a light headache. If that's not proof enough that this stuff is toxic to a clean and detoxed body, I don't know what is. Also, keep in mind that doctors recommend their patients that have high blood pressure to reduce salt in their diet.

In an article published in *Living Nutrition*, Volume 18, David Klein, Ph.D. advises to avoid all salt, because:

> It's a toxic, irritating, corrosive, stimulating, enervating and potentially deadly poison...These inorganic substances may be trendy but they are not healthful. In addition to sodium chloride, they contain numerous toxic elements including heavy metals such as aluminum, cadmium, lead and mercury. These wreak havoc in the body, and are difficult to eliminate.

If you live in a northern region or near the ocean, you have probably seen how rock salt and salt spray eats steel members and chrome coatings on automobiles. If you've ever had an open flesh wound and exposed it to salt, your senses will have told you how destructive it is. Salt paralyzes the intestinal villi and kills cells—would you knowingly bathe your delicate villi, your arteries, veins and capillaries with such a corrosive solution? Salt brine kills insects and "pickles" vegetables. Do you want to run a solution of that through your brain 24 hours a day? An ounce of salt, taken all at once, spells suicide.

You cannot become healthy if your sense of taste is befuddled by unnatural flavorings. Salt does not bring out the flavor of food; it overpowers your taste buds, numbing them to all sensation other than additional salt, causing unnatural cravings, overeating and beverage guzzling.

Salt bonds with water, and its toxicity necessitates extra fluid intake. The body's dilution response causes the cells to become dehydrated, severely impairing health. Salt also throws off the blood's electrolyte balance (e.g., the sodium to potassium ratio) and acidifies the body, eroding health and impeding healing.

Most illnesses cannot be overcome when salt is part of the diet...

Hypertension (high blood pressure), edema, cardiovascular disease, stroke, atherosclerosis, asthma, arthritis, rheumatism, Alzheimer's disease, lupus, premenstrual syndrome, gout, cancer, and a host of other disease causations are linked to salt. Can the body handle a little bit of salt? Maybe, but not on a regular basis.

We use mineral salts in our daily lives, but its alternative, plant foods, are the natural answer. Fruits and vegetables and/or liquids from them contain all the mineral salts we need, in safe, organic, bio-available, and usable forms.

Sugar and its substitutes

There are tons of different forms of sugar available on the supermarket shelves. You may even have some of these (or all of them) in your pantry right now! But it's important to understand the differences between table sugar, honey, artificial sweeteners, and high-fructose corn syrup when it comes to how each of them affect your body. Processed sugar is well-known to contribute to inflammation, decrease the strength of your immune system, and increase your risk of living with significant health conditions such as heart disease, diabetes, metabolic syndrome, and even cancer.

Before the 1900s, when Americans were estimated to ingest only five pounds of sugar each year, it was rare to see diagnoses of diabetes, heart disease, and cancer. Fast forward to today, and the average American ingests over 135 pounds a year—which marks an incredible increase of 27 times the average consumption of sugar.

According to Dr. Isaac Eliaz, MD, MS, LAc: "Forms of sugar that are not processed are better choices than highly processed and refined sugars, for several reasons. Highly refined sugars tend to produce a much higher spike in blood glucose levels than do unprocessed or unrefined sugars. They also lack in trace nutrients that can still be found in unrefined, more natural sugars." It's very hard for your body to process sugars that have been highly refined. As a result, your nutrients are steadily depleted as your body tries to restore balance once these toxins have been ingested.

The best choice would be to just eat fresh fruits (one type of fruit at a time, preferably). You don't have to worry about sugar in fruits, because it gets metabolized differently. (Although, if you have diabetes or candida, you should be careful of any kind of sweet stuff. If you don't know how to properly combine foods while on a fruitarian diet, you could end up making your health condition worse.) It is very important to know that it's not about how much sugar you consume (I am talking about sugar in fruits), but about how much sugar is in your bloodstream at a given point of time. For example, if you eat watermelon for breakfast, you can eat the entire watermelon and be fine—even if you have diabetes or systemic candida (please, don't try any radical changes in your diet at home without proper supervision, especially if you have diabetes or systemic candida).

In my personal experience, I was able to cure colitis and systemic candida with a mono-fruitarian diet. I had an experienced supervisor and teacher who was a fruitarian himself for over 26 years who had an extended experience in this department. He healed himself from 74 different allergies, IBS, and other health issues, as well as helped thousands of patients in the past few decades. He taught me about the rules of properly combining fruits in order not to have too much sugar in my bloodstream.

On a proper fruitarian diet you don't have to count calories, nor limit your intake of fruits. Please, keep in mind that if you poorly combine your fruits, for example avocado (high fat content) and banana (high glycemic load), you are looking for getting your systemic candida and/or other health conditions worse, instead of better. If you don't know the rules of a fruitatian diet, you might make yourself sicker than when you were on a regular diet. This is the reason why people quite often claim that they tried a fruitarian diet, and it either didn't work or it made them sicker. If you are doing something you don't know about, but still want to achieve good results, it's best to do it under the supervision of an expert (or not do it at all).

For natural sweeteners, I would suggest raw honey or raw organic powdered Stevia. Just keep in mind that even though honey is considered to be a superfood, it is not vegan. Stevia comes in a green super sweet powder and a little goes a long way. As a sweetener, you can also use dates for recipes and smoothies or your own homemade coconut or almond milk. Dates are number one on my list for sweeteners. After you rid your body of addictive substances such as refined sugars, the cravings will subside and you can better appreciate foods that are naturally sweet on their own.

What do you shower with? What do you use for lotions and makeup? What do you brush your teeth with?

When I started learning about toxicity, it took me months to change everything that I used to use for new stuff that didn't have toxins, or at least was the most "natural" and with the least amount of additives. It took me even longer to psychologically adjust to all the changes I have made. It took a lot of experimenting to find what was working specifically for me.

When I took my shampoo bottle and started researching each ingredient individually by putting their name into Google (I would use the name of ingredient combined with word "toxicity"), I was in shock. For example, one of the ingredients on my old shampoo bottle was phenoxyethanol. I took my time to sit in front of my computer and look up "Phenoxyethanol toxicity." The info that came up was terrifying.

Phenoxyethanol is the new darling of the chemical industry and is increasingly turning up in cosmetics as an alternative preservative to parabens. It only recently came to public attention in the US when the FDA issued a warning about its use in a cream, called Mommy Bliss, for nursing mothers. The FDA **warned** that phenoxyethanol can cause a shutdown of the central nervous system, vomiting, and contact dermatitis. So, what is phenoxyethanol, and is it really safer than parabens or should we try to avoid it?

Phenoxyethanol is a glycol ether. A glycol is a chemical that can be found in many household items (such as lacquer or paint) and even some uncommon ones (like jet fuel). In cosmetics, phenoxyethanol acts as an antibacterial agent. You can also find phenoxyethanol in perfume as a stabilizer. If you look up the MSDS safety sheet, you'll see that phenoxyethanol is labelled as harmful when swallowed, inhaled, or absorbed through the skin (and that it can also result in reproductive damage). Of course, the MSDS is talking about concentrations that are 100% phenoxyethanol. Wouldn't it be safe in small quantities? For example, cosmetics usually have a concentration of between 0.5%–1%.

Animal studies have been conducted that show that phenoxyethanol is a toxic substance that causes harm to the brain and nervous system when absorbed in a moderate concentration. Japan limits the amount that can be included in cosmetics. The European Union has labelled phenoxyethanol as a skin irritant when applied in low doses (a fact that scientific studies support). Data sheets from the Environmental Protection Agency (EPA) discuss testing results in mice that show genetic mutations, chromosomal changes, reproductive disruptions, and testicular atrophy.

There are reports of medical professionals who have contracted allergies as a result of phenoxyethanol. In fact, there are more than 3,000 known allergens—and a research team in Germany ranked phenoxyethanol as one of the top ten. An Italian study also deemed phenoxyethanol as an allergan, while the Journal of the American College of Toxicology reports it as a mild skin irritant in rabbits.

Before the FDA took note, a German research team concluded that phenoxyethanol could potentially be a neurotoxin. In the body, this chemical is broken down into phenol and acetaldehyde, the former of which can inhibit the primary response mechanism of your immune system. Interestingly enough (and perhaps even more concerning), phenoxyethanol is utilized as an anti-bacterial agent in vaccines. The second byproduct of phenoxyethanol, acetaldehyde, is a potential carcinogen, with studies showing that it can irritate the respiratory tract, skin, and eyes.

Given the wealth of evidence, I'd rather pass on it even at concentrations of 1% or lower. Also, keep in mind, this preservative is used in makeup, shampoos, conditioners, and lotions—which is basically everything you have in your bathroom cabinet. Are you even sure that you are still staying under that 1% mark? If you use more lotion, such as all over your body, does it measure at 2%, 3%, or higher?

I actually took my time and went over each ingredient on each bottle of every product I used at that time and learned about each additive, chemical, and preservative they put in the products I used to use. I realized that we are using a cocktail of lethal toxic substances every day. No matter how small a quantity you use (for example, drinking just a tiny bit of "gasoline" a day), you are going to be affected by it sooner or later. It's the accumulative effect in the end that matters. After researching, I tossed away all the expensive and fashionable (yet toxic) stuff I used. It was time to find clean and organic products without additives or with additives that won't make my body cells mutate. I didn't want to have all the bouquet of "wonderful" effects of health destruction that you would gain from using expensive commercial products.

Our society conditions us to compete, so we work for our own choice of poison. We have to work for all that is considered "best" (i.e., expensive and fashionable), so we can earn enough money to buy our own poison that we falsely believe we need. The fact that it's slowly killing us is irrelevant. Just because it didn't happen instantly after its use today makes us aasume that it is not harmful. Some of the products can actually appear to be making a temporary fix (at least you might think so on external level). You might see cosmetics smoothen wrinkles after applying some eye cream, but in all actuality, a cocktail of toxins gets absorbed into your cells, such as neurotoxins and carcinogens.

My father always told me that it is OK to eat a little poison (like what we find in food preservatives, or fashionable lotions), as our bodies are designed to deal with it. However, when I look at my father—a man in his 60s, with terrible undereye darkness (a sign that his liver is not working properly) and other various sorts of health issues, including blood pressure, anxiety, tumors/cysts under his skin, and the suspicion of prostate cancer—I highly doubt that his theory of eating everything and using everything in moderation works.

As a millionaire who always buys "the best of the best," my father is still just a human and can't escape the results of improper eating. His wife always spends a lot of money "maintaining" herself by doing all sorts of toxic procedures, masks, and applying the "best" lotions for face. She always ate the "best" foods that millions of dollars can buy. Unfortunately, she had to battle cancer and was not even 60 years old when she started falling apart health-wise. What a high price to pay for "fashion" and the "best lotions, and creams, and foods, and all that wonderful stuff" that my father's money could buy! The only thing money *can't* buy is your health.

As David Wolfe wrote in one of his books: "If you want to take advice from someone, just make sure you want to end up like them in regards to aging, health, and looks."

I researched a lot of different lotions and you can find a huge variety of organic lotions where they use beeswax as emulsifier, and not even one toxic ingredient. I was delighted by those choices. However, I was looking for simplicity: for me, less is more. So, I personally settled on pure organic cold-pressed almond oil for my body. I also use organic cold-pressed cucumber or jojoba oil for my face.

I looked for a long time into many other face treatment items that we are taught to use (like cleanser or toner), and I realized that it's all just bogus. We are what we eat. If you are clean on the inside, your pores are not enlarged, and you don't get blackheads, pimples, or any other problems with your skin. All the face treatments that you are investing in are not helping the problems. All that they will do is suppress the symptoms of the issue without fixing the real problem that gets worse and worse each day. After all, everyone is trying to sell you something. A lot of things are just not necessary. As a matter of fact, once I got on a simple program for my face and body maintenance, I started looking 10 years younger in a matter of six months. I was very surprised, as I always thought that without all that expensive stuff I used, my skin would age faster. On the contrary, the cleaner I got (in reference to my diet), I saw progressively amazing, age-defying results.

I rinse my face with just water. I don't use any cleanser (but you can, there are a ton of organic alternatives that don't have even one bad ingredient). Then, I use astringent which I make myself. I take Witch Hazel, add a little bit of rose water, a few drops of organic rosemary oil, a few drops of tea tree oil, and a few drops of peppermint oil, and it's done. It's very inexpensive, and it goes a long way. I use it only once a day, in the evening, after being exposed to outdoor pollution.

For shampoo and conditioner, I found a great solution, and it is the closest to "clean" and non-toxic that I found. I use Soap Nuts/Soap Berry Shampoo from NaturOli (it's a shampoo and conditioner in one). It works for me, but it might not work on processed hair. You might have to look for a conditioner until you grow out your natural hair (if that's what you intend on doing). Or you can use coconut oil (rub it in the scalp and on your hair, leave it in for an hour, and then wash it out with Soap Nuts). I also use NaturOli 100% Natural Hair Serum Anti-Frizz, Smoothing Detangler for my hair.

There are many layers of "healthy." For example, whole cooked foods are better then McDonalds, but raw foods are better then cooked foods and so on. Well, it's the same with products you choose to use for your skin and hair. When I started the search, I wanted the simplest products and I found alternatives for shampoos and conditioners. You can use plain baking soda for shampoo, and vinegar for conditioner. You can find tons of online recipes on how to mix it and what to add to make it work specifically for your hair.

I also learned that even if you want to change your hair color, you don't need to put chemicals in it. The closest to "natural" would be henna for red color, indigo for black color, and lemon juice for blonde color (or blonde highlights). You can find a lot of different variations of recipes online as well.

For armpits, I realized how toxic deodorant is. It is widely offered, and even potassium alum (naturally occurring) is very, very questionable and—in my opinion, based on my research—toxic. So, I found the solution: I use baking soda (one teaspoon for a cup of water) with a few drops of peppermint essential oil. It does magic for me. There are other alternatives as well, such as lemon juice and vinegar.

Although, I should mention that this transition took me some time as I was not used to sweating (the armpit deodorants that we are familiar with using block the sweat glands, so you always have dry armpits), but if we can't sweat, we can't get rid of toxins. It was very weird at the beginning when I switched to baking soda. I went back and forth a few times before I psychologically accepted this change.

The change was the constant sensation of "wet" from sweating. With time, I got used to the new feeling of being able to sweat and detox through my underarms. Also, when I did the longest fast of my life (35 days of water fast) followed by a 100% mono-fruitarian diet, I realized that my sweat doesn't smell any longer, and I stopped using anything in my underarms altogether.

For my teeth, I used 1.5% diluted food-grade peroxide for rinsing my mouth and keeping my teeth white. But once I switched from vegan raw diet to 100% frutarian, I stopped it all together. My teeth were clean and white on the fruit diet by themselves, all without any help. As toothpaste, I used four drops of coconut oil with one drop of tea tree oil. Coconut oil whitens your teeth and kills the bacteria along with tea tree oil. When I switched to just oils, it felt weird at first, but I stuck with it. Later, when I tried to go back to "regular" toothpaste, I realized that it was too abrasive for me, and way too toxic as well. Of course, I looked up the toxicity of every ingredient in the toothpaste I used at that time and came to the realization that it's all no good. Later, when I switched from a vegan raw diet to a 100% fruitarian diet, I just used a toothbrush without anything on it and it seemed to be working just fine.

For makeup, I found the site www.100percentpure.com, where you can get non-toxic products. There are also a lot of options on Etsy, the website where people create their own small businesses with their unique, handmade, clean products. Whatever you are looking for, you will find the answer online. The question is: do you need it? And why do you need it? I just mentioned a few alternatives to thousands of possibilities of what you can be using. For all I know, you can be using only fresh fruits and vegetables for your skin, face, and hair. I know some people who do that. Also, when you are completely detoxed, you don't stink when you sweat, nor do you have morning breath, and your hair doesn't get dirty as fast. Therefore, at a much further stage of detoxing, you won't need a deodorant, or possibly any shampoo. At that point, your sweat is going to smell like sweet fruits by itself, and maybe you will need to wash your hair twice a month with a little baking soda. The more we detox and come to the natural state, the less we need.

What to use best: glass or plastic bottle?

When bottling water, make sure you use glass (dark amber glass, if possible). We now know that plastic is non-biodegradable; instead, it is photodegradable, which means that the plastic particles begin to leach off into the water upon contact with light. Plastic in the human body is one of the leading causes for hormone disruptions, endocrine problems, and arthritic conditions. Plastics create what is known as xenoestrogens that deposit themselves into our fat cells. This leads to an extreme imbalance of the hormone estrogen. This has been shown to create an over-feminization in men, where excess belly fat and even breast development appears. Women run a serious risk of increased chances of certain types of cancer by producing imbalanced estrogen dominance, especially synthetic xenoestrogens.

Glass or plastic: this seemingly small detail seems to affect your entire life, so the next time you go to buy water, don't worry about paying a little extra for a glass bottle instead of plastic. You will win much more in the long run. Also, remember that toxicity is an accumulative process and it takes just a tiny bit at a time to get to a landfill of filth that is built up in your body day after day, which will cause detrimental damage to your health in the long run.

The microwave oven

Your health is directly tied to the quality of foods that you eat. The old adage, "You are what you eat" has never been more true. And perhaps there's room to add the way that food is prepared—and the sacrifices that we make for convenience. Microwave ovens may be able to quickly heat up a meal, but there is a high cost to your health attached to that expediency. Even putting green beans or broccoli florets into the microwave for a quick zap could have serious consequences. The way that microwave ovens work is by tearing apart the molecules within your food, making some nutrients completely useless and even carcinogenic.

It's also worth mentioning that microwaving food that is wrapped in plastic or paper can be just as harmful. Toxic chemicals are used to create packaging for pizza, popcorn, and many other microwaveable foods. As reported by Nutrition Action Newsletter in 1990, this includes toluene, benzene, xylene, and polyethylene terpthalate. When these types of foods are microwaved in a plastic container, toxins are released into your food. This includes BPA, a compound that is similar to estrogen and is widely used in plastic. Many dishes that are microwave-safe include BPA.

The molecular distortion that comes from microwaving is not limited to food. In 1991, after receiving a transfusion of blood that had been microwaved (transfusions typically require blood warming first), an Oklahoma woman died. The $30M lawsuit, *Warner vs. Hillcrest Medical Center*, was highly publicized.

I dare you to test the theory of how detrimental the microwaves are. Just buy two cheap, but strong, identical plants, bring them home, and put them in the best spot in your house for them to prosper. Then, each time you water them, water one plant with the sink water, and the other with microwaved water. If those plants are of the same kind, they should be doing equally well, provided microwaved water doesn't cause any harm. To your surprise, you will find that the plant that you watered with microwaved water, would have perished within one to two weeks. The damage would be irreversible.

Now, our human tissue gets the effects of the same damage, but because we have many more cells to spare than plants, we don't die right away. Instead, we deteriorate slowly (it's an accumulative effect). People come to false conclusions: they think that if they didn't die right away from using the microwave (and by eating microwaved foods), then it's OK. However, in reality, they are destroying their health one little step at a time.

Microwaves leak radiation, and the FDA—or any other organization that states they are safe—is giving you the misinformation for the glory of appliance sales and moving the economy. Even when the microwave oven is not working, it is leaking radiation at all times. If they tell you that it's not a dangerous amount, then please explain to me what that means? If I will be feeding gasoline to a child in micro amounts, the child won't die and he/she won't get sick right away—which, by FDA standards, it must mean that it's safe, right? But if I do it continuously, the child will eventually get very sick and possibly die from the sickness that they have developed. It is the same thing with microwaves. The radiation from the waves can travel through the walls. There is no escape from it. Keep in mind that standing a foot away from a microwave while it is running can expose you to upwards of 400 milliGauss. A mere 4 milliGauss has been firmly linked to causing leukemia. Thus, it would certainly be wise to avoid exposure to microwave oven all together.

Once I learned all this, and watched on YouTube how one person measured radiation around microwave (which was a way higher then it was supposed to be despite standing at the other end of the kitchen across from it), I threw away my microwave oven for good. Don't feel sorry to toss away something that is damaging your system. You will lose much more if you keep the harmful item in the house. Doctors are very expensive, and saving your health from damage is priceless.

It is good to remember that it is best to eat all your food raw without using anything to heat it up—but if you do choose to use some way of heating and cooking your food up, I would recommend choosing the least damaging cookware that doesn't leak toxic material (most cheap frying pans and pots do). Search "Waterless Cookware" on the Internet to see product information. It is not cheap (a 15-piece set will cost you around $200), but it will save you a lot on doctor's bills in long run. It is a great investment if you prefer to stick with cooked foods.

The damage from wearing bras: The link between breast cancer and bras

I would highly recommend reading the book: *Dressed to Kill: The Link between Breast Cancer and Bras* by Sydney Ross Singer and Soma Grismaijer. Singer and Grismaijer have collected striking evidence that bra-wearing may be a major risk factor associated with breast cancer. Women who wear tight-fitting bras 24 hours a day are 125 times more likely to have breast cancer than women who do not wear bras at all. Their interpretation is that tight clothing inhibits the proper functioning of the lymphatic system (an internal network of vessels and nodes that flushes wastes from the body) and leads to a buildup of carcinogenic compounds in the constricted areas. According to the authors:

When Soma and I did our research for *Dressed to Kill*, we were not aware of how easily women can recover from fibrocystic breast disease by foregoing the bra. Bras, by their very design, alter the shape of the breasts for fashion. To alter breast shape you have to apply constant pressure on the breast tissue. That is why bras are elastic garments. This pressure from the bra impedes the circulation in the breast tissue, specifically, the circulation of the lymphatic system.

This system is composed of microscopic vessels that originate in the breast tissue and drain the tissue of fluid, which is directed through these vessels to the lymph nodes. The lymphatic vessels are extremely thin and small, and have no pump, such as the heart, to propel its contents forward. As a result, lymphatic vessels are easily constricted by external pressure, such as that applied to the breast tissue constantly by the brassiere. It is compression of these lymph vessels that prevents the proper draining of the breast tissue, leading to fluid accumulation in the breast. Medically, this is called lymphedema of the breast, secondary to constriction from the bra.

This fluid accumulation leads to breast tenderness and pain, and ultimately the fluid develops into cysts. The cysts over time become hard, and we have a picture of the creation of fibrocystic breast disease. Within days or weeks of ending breast constriction by bras, the breast tissue is allowed to flush out this excess fluid, cysts disappear, and breast pain and tenderness are minimal if at all present.

From our research with hundreds of women, getting rid of the bra has resulted in remarkable recovery of breast health in over 95% of the cases. Since foregoing the bra for a month is cost-free, risk-free, and may prove beneficial, we encourage all women who wear bras to partake in a self-study to see for themselves, on themselves, whether their bras have been damaging their breasts.

Keep in mind that breast disease is only a problem in bra wearing cultures. Women who are bra-free have the same breast cancer incidence as men. And don't wait for the cancer detection and treatment industry to endorse this information before you try it. Billions of dollars are made each year treating breast cancer. Nobody will make money by women loosening up to prevent this disease. The prevention of breast disease is up to each individual woman. Just stop binding the breasts with bras in the name of fashion, and begin to love yourself and respect your body.

In the book, it explains that if you use a "crutch" like a bra, your muscles that support your breasts would atrophy, so eventually, you won't have any support of your own. But, given enough time and little exercise, you can bring your natural muscle support back and feel awesome. I highly recommend you to try this experiment for health's sake if you read the above-mentioned book.

Flu shots

It's pretty much a given that, if you get a flu shot these days, you will immediately get sick. Here is the problem: most people don't even know what the flu is. I will try to make this easy for you to understand. Let's start at the beginning.

- A **cold** is when the natural bacteria of the body goes in and feeds on tissue that has been damaged by toxicity. So a cold is a good thing. It doesn't need to be "cured." It's your own body's toxicity that needs to be cured.

- A **flu virus** is a solvent that the body creates internally. This happens when the body's bacteria is unable to break down its own toxic waste because of inorganic substances like heavy metals, pesticides, and food additives. In other words, the body has become so toxic that the natural bacteria (the cold) is getting killed when it tries to eat away our toxic tissues. The virus mixes with water (the main solvent on our planet) and goes into the cells and washes away the toxic elements without damaging the integrity of the cell itself (to allow it to maintain functionality). In this way, think of the flu like detergent in your washing machine, cleaning the dirt off your clothes.

- A **virus** is not alive. There is no nucleus, no circulatory system, no digestive system, etc. Saying that a virus is alive is like saying the soap in your shower is alive.

- Viruses are produced by the **cells in the body**, so they are specific to certain types of tissue in the body. In other words, your body will create one virus to clean out the blood and a different virus to clean out the lymphatic system.

- Viruses **do not jump across species**. You CANNOT "catch" a virus. Swine and avian viruses are specific to swine and avian tissue. The only way to get swine or avian tissue in YOUR blood is to have it injected into YOUR blood.

- **All viruses are good viruses**. All colds are good colds. Without the two we would drown in our own toxins and die from toxic shock.

Flu shots don't work. At this point, hopefully you are asking yourself: why do they even exist? What are they really injecting into you? Why do most people get sick immediately after getting flu shots? People wouldn't be getting sick in the first place if they were not toxic.

To create the seasonal flu vaccine, flu strains are selected and then cultivated within chick embryos. After a few weeks, they are infused with formaldehyde (a known cancer-inducing agent) and become inactive. Thimerosal, a known cancer-causing agent that contains 49% mercury by weight, is then added as a preservative. Why would a cancer-causing agent be included in a vaccine? Plenty of healthcare professionals are asking themselves the same thing. And the CDC reports that most flu vaccines use thimerosal as the preservative, with some containing over 250 times the safety limit for mercury ingestion as lsited by the EPA.

By now, most people are well aware that children and fetuses are most at risk of damage from this neurotoxin, as their brains are still developing. Yet the CDC still recommends that children over six months, and pregnant women, receive the flu vaccine each year. In addition to mercury, flu vaccines also contain 63 other toxic or hazardous ingredients. I will not cite all of them, but I will give an example:

- Aluminum – a neurotoxin that has been linked to Alzheimer's disease
- Triton X-100 – a detergent
- Phenol (carbolic acid)
- Ethylene glycol (antifreeze)
- Betapropiolactone – a disinfectant
- Nonoxynol – used to kill or stop growth of STDs
- Octoxinol 9 – a vaginal spermicide
- Sodium phosphate

How safe are vaccines? Before 1985, people were only getting three vaccines (DPT, MMR, and Polio). Each individual virus is called an antigen. Now there are 16 vaccines and there are multiple doses of all 16 of those. The difference is that if you added all those vaccine antigens back then—like MMRs (three vaccine antigens with one shot), DPT (three vaccine antigens with one shot), and polio (it has actually three viruses in them, so you get three different viruses in one shot)—it would result in a total of nine vaccine antigens.

If you add up the sum of all total antigens that children got before 1985, they got 33 antigens injected into them before they started kindergarten.

Up through 2010, they got up to 156 vaccine antigens injected into children before they even started kindergarten. Even more vaccines have been added since then. There are measurable amounts of chemicals and milligram amounts of gelatin in MMR and the chicken pox vaccine. In addition, there are 63 different types of chemicals in those vaccines.

Not all vaccines have those 63 chemicals, but if you get all the vaccines, you get all 63 different types of chemicals—some of which are known carcinogens, some are known to cause asthma...the list is endless.

Mercury is absent from most vaccines, but it's not out of all of them. It's still in multi-dose flu shots that they start giving infants at six months of age, and they get them every year through out their life. So, you are still getting doses of mercury. There is also tons of aluminum—and when I say tons, I mean milligram amounts. That is measurable amounts, not little trace amounts. Babies get about 88 milligrams of mercury injected into them if they got all doses of the mercury-laden vaccines. And the government goes: "Whoops, somebody forgot to do the math..."

So, back in 2004, when the issue became clear, the government didn't tell the pharmaceutical industry to pull off all those vaccines and re-make them. They said: "When you make new ones, just replace the mercury." When the mercury problem became a really big issue (and yes, it did become a big deal), it was not just the mercury. It was aluminum and other chemicals that are present in all these vaccine antigens, all these viruses and bacteria, stray viruses that are known to cause cancer, and all kinds of toxic mixtures inside vaccines. Most of the parents as well as physicians, that never bothered to read the package, think that all that is in there is a little bit of sterile water, a little bit of attenuated or killed virus, and that's it. How can it hurt you?

I would strongly recommend asking your physician for the "package insert" of the vaccine that you consider getting for yourself or for your child. I would recommend to carefully study all side effects of that vaccine, and then make an informed decision if you wish to get vaccinated. For example, Tripedia Vaccine "side effects" are acknowledged by the FDA. Here is what the "package insert" of Tripedia says:

"Adverse effects reported during post-approval use of Tripedia vaccine include idiopathic thrombocytopenic purpura, SIDS [that means SUDDEN INFANT DEATH SYNDROME], anaphylactic reaction [that means sudden, widespread, potentially severe and life-threatening allergic reactions], cellulitis, autism [that means you are risking getting brain damage after getting this vaccine], convulsion/grand mal convulsion, encephalopathy, hypotonia, neuropathy, somnolence and aphea. Events were included in this list above, because of the seriousness or frequency of reporting."

All I urge you to do is to carefully read the insert on each and every vaccine you are planning on getting to make the informed decision if you need it.

Personally, I feel that I don't want any amount of heavy metals, carcinogens or toxins in my body—so just based on that alone, I can't submit myself to vaccinations. I also was "lucky" that due to my severe allergies through out my life (before I became raw vegan and started detoxing my system), I was exempt from any vaccinations due to the possibility of severe adverse reactions. Because my mother was a doctor, and realized that any vaccine might literally take my life, she always had a way of getting all the needed paperwork to excuse me from those mandatory vaccinations throughout my life. As an adult, I would never intentionally go and pump my system with all sorts of toxic matter that comes together with that vaccine and damage my health. I believe that if you are not toxic, you will not get sick no matter what. It's just a matter of cleansing and detoxing your system—which, in my opinion, contradicts injecting heavy metals and toxins in your body, even if it's in micro amounts.

What do you drink?

I learned, unfortunately, that our tap water in the US is not suitable for drinking. I believe it's not even suitable for showering, unless it has been filtered. Not everyone can afford the luxury of filtered water, but the question is: is that really necessary?

After the Fukushima accident, the water (as well as the environment) in the US is radioactive (a fact which is kept hush-hush). There is a huge mixture of pharmaceuticals, microscopic fecal matter, toxic materials, heavy metals, chlorine, and fluoride in American water.

Fluoride is a carcinogen that leads to cancer development in the body (through an accumulative process that takes years). It's a poison that accumulates in our bones. It has been associated with cancer in young males, osteoporosis, reduced I.Q., and hip fractures in the elderly, to name a few. The mechanism by which fluoride's lethal poisoning of man and animals occurs is presented. "Low" level fluoridation of municipal water exhibits well-known alterations in teeth and bone structure and calcification of tendons and ligaments. "Moderate" doses cause spinal deformities, increased hip fractures, and kidney and gallstones (if fluoride exposure is sufficiently high or prolonged). "Higher" levels cause death and are responsible for its major industrial use as a rodenticide.

Dr. Paul Connett is a trained chemist and a specialist in environmental chemistry. He says: "Water fluoridation is a very bad medicine, because once you put it in the water, you can't control the dose. You can't control who gets it. There is no oversight. You're allowing a community to do to everyone what a doctor can do to no one, i.e. force a patient to take a particular medication."

Community-wide fluoridation in the US began in 1945. Before that time, fluoride was listed as a toxin in the Journal of the American Dental Association and the Journal of the American Medical Association. They claimed that fluroide concentrations of 1ppm was just as toxic as arsenic and lead and that fluoride disrupts cell permeability, respectively. And in 1944, the American Dental Association said that "Drinking water containing as little as 1.2 ppm fluoride will cause developmental disturbances." Even if you are drinking filtered water, you are likely still ingesting fluoride through procesesed or canned food, since fluoridated water is part of the preparation process.

Fluoride builds up in the pineal gland and causes calcification. Germans used fluoride on prisoners to make them docile and obedient. When the pineal gland is calcified, you can't be fully yourself (you become more like a robot that takes orders without questioning, and that makes it easy to control the public). Awesome abilities such as telepathy, clairvoyance, remote viewing, and other extraordinary abilities are inter-connected with the activation of the pineal gland (no wonder we don't believe in any of these abilities; if our pineal glands are calcified, we never get to express and/or experience them).

Another chemical to be avoided at all times is chlorine. Inhaling steamed water can cause lung cancer from inhaling the chlorine that is evaporating from it. Chlorine is also carcinogenic and it works best if you have prolonged exposure to it. For example, when you shower every day with chlorinated water, and if it's hot water, you can inhale chlorine through steam. You brush your teeth with it, or each time you wash a fruit or vegetable—and even your own hands—you are soaking them with chemicals.

Another issue is that our septic system is set in such a way that it recycles used water, so all that water that has been used to flush excrement, tampons, and urine, is re-used. Most Americans are on some kind of pharmaceutical aid, which in itself is a huge medical corporate business that makes millions of dollars from the population. A lot of pharmaceutical waste is excreted through human urine and it gets back into our system. Filtration systems are not effective against micro-fecal matter, micro-particles from used tampons, or traces of pharmaceuticals. That is why they need to add a lot of chlorine to kill most of the bacteria. They add other deadly toxins like fluoride and then provide us with the result: water that is ready for you to use to shower, drink, or use for cooking.

The solution for this problem is to install a filtration system for the entire house where you live. This will limit your exposure to all unwanted toxins. There are RO (Reverse Osmosis) filters that can be installed in the whole house. There are also filters that can structure your water on top of RO water, and that would be the best combination. Structured water will hydrate your body much better than any other water. I usually put my drinking water out in the sun (to sun-charge) and structure my water. I also use a glass jar with a glass lid for it.

In addition to this, there are also all sorts of less expensive charcoal filters that don't really remove fluoride or heavy metals, but remove most of chlorine. So, do your research and find the best filter for the right price that will work for you. If you can't afford a filtration system, there is still another solution. You can buy RO water at any health store; it costs 35 cents per gallon in the US. They also sell 5-gallon glass jugs for you to get your water. (Note: I am not sure if this is accurate, but I also read that RO water is radiation-free, as the RO filter filters the radiation out.)

I am not going into the discussion of drinking anything else but water, because I believe it's common sense. Anything that is mixed in a bottle and processed with added sugar is not good for you. If you want fresh juice, you have to juice it yourself, preferably from organic fruits. All the mixed drinks at the store are heavily processed and pasteurized (through heating, all the nutrients and healthy enzymes are killed, and only sugar and toxins are left behind) and they are damaging for your health, as store-bought juices contain fluoride and other toxins.

I also believe that everyone knows that drinking pop or soda is not the best idea. Coca-Cola and Pepsi are used as pesticides by Indian farmers. Phosphoric acid, for example, is highly acidic and may function as a pest deterrent. Perhaps it's the aspartame in the diet soda. Since aspartame is well known to promote neurological side effects in humans, it is conceivable that it may function as a neurotoxic pesticide when sprayed on crops. In addition to being useful as pesticides when sprayed on crops, Coke and Pepsi are also very good at cleaning up blood stains from concrete, due to their carbonation effect. They can also clean toilet bowls, car bumpers, and garage floors as well. Oh, and if you really want to challenge your health, you can also drink Coke and Pepsi—although that is not advisable unless you really want a stomach full of high-fructose corn syrup. (And don't forget that 99% of corn is GMO in the US, which means that your high-fructose corn syrup is even more damaging to your body.)

Are humans carnivores or herbivores?

It might feel as though meat has always been a part of our diet, even since the very beginning of man. But historically speaking, we haven't been eating meat for very long at all. Dr. T. Colin Campbell, professor emeritus at Cornell University and author of *The China Study*, says that: "The birth of agriculture only started about 10,000 years ago, at a time when it became considerably more convenient to herd animals. This is not nearly as long as the time [that] fashioned our basic biochemical functionality (at least tens of millions of years) and which functionality depends on the nutrient composition of plant-based foods."

There's some agreement on that. In his book, *The Power of Your Plate*, Dr. Neal Barnard says: "Early humans had diets very much like other great apes, which is to say a largely plant-based diet, drawing on foods we can pick with our hands. Research suggests that meat-eating probably began by scavenging, eating the leftovers that carnivores had left behind. However, our bodies have never adapted to it. To this day, meat-eaters have a higher incidence of heart disease, cancer, diabetes, and other problems."

Even one of the highest, most authoritative figures in paleontology echoes this idea that man was designed to be a herbivore, not a carnivore. Paleontologist Dr. Richard Leakey states that,"[you] can't tear flesh by hand.... We wouldn't have been able to deal with food source that required those large canines." Of course, we do have "canine" teeth, but these are nothing compared to the teeth of actual carnivores—like, say, a tiger or a wolf.

And our hands don't have sharp talons or points in which to take down our prey. Instead, our hands are just the right shape— with the perfect range of functionality—to pick up fruits and vegetables from the ground, from bushes, and from trees. Another interesting thought is the length of our intestines. Carnivores tend to have short intestinal tracts, so as to get rid of any meat as quickly as possible. In contrast, ours are much longer, similar to the intestinal tracts of other herbivores. Most importantly, for the most part, we don't really have that internal instinct that would push us to run after prey, kill them, and immediately dive in to eat.

Ultimately, although we might have eaten some meat here and there when we were hunting and gathering, it wasn't a regular staple. And there's no reason why it should be now. Dr. William C. Roberts, editor of the American Journal of Cardiology, echoes this sentiment: "Although we think we are, and we act as if we are, human beings are not natural carnivores. When we kill animals to eat them, they end up killing us, because their flesh, which contains cholesterol and saturated fat, was never intended for human beings, who are natural herbivores."

Meat isn't good for us. Eating meat gives us lower energy levels, makes us sleep more, and puts us at higher risk for serious diseases such as cancer, diabetes, heart disease, and obesity. But if you're used to having meat as part of your everyday diet, it's hard to make that switch—after all, habits die hard. And there's a lot of propaganda that we've been fed about why eating meat is so beneficial, such as getting protein from meat and dairy. I've been there, too. Now that I look back at it, I think that I was very attached to the way that I was brought up, and the traditions that were connected to those meals. For example, we always eat turkey for Thanksgiving, and our family always did ham for Christmas and Easter. Those meals were tied directly to laughter, happiness, family bonding, and togetherness. How could I give up those decades-old traditions? There's no denying that those emotions and my memories of the foods we ate are deeply intertwined.

But making that switch from a carnivore diet to an herbivore diet is crucial to your long-term health. There are plenty of experienced nutritional scientists and anthropologists that support the idea that humans are designed to be herbivores—and that we will be much healthier if we stop eating meat.

Let's take a deeper look at this and compare the physiological traits of carnivores, herbivores, and omnivores and see where human beings fit in.

Facial Muscles

- **Carnivore**: Reduced to allow wide mouth gape
- **Herbivore**: Well-developed
- **Omnivore**: Reduced
- **Human**: Well-developed

Sweat

- **Meat-eaters**: Have no skin pores and perspire through the tongue
- **Herbivores**: Perspire through skin pores
- **Humans**: Perspire through skin pores

Meat-eating animals hunt in the cool of the night and sleep during the day when it is hot, so they do not need sweat glands to cool their bodies. That means they do not perspire through their skin; instead, they sweat through their tongues. On the other hand, vegetarian animals, such as cows, horses, zebras, deer, etc., spend most of their time in the sun gathering their food and they freely perspire through their skin to cool their bodies.

Jaw Type

- **Carnivore**: Angle not expanded
- **Herbivore:** Expanded angle
- **Omnivore**: Angle not expanded
- **Human**: Expanded angle

Jaw Joint Location

- **Carnivore**: On same plane as molar teeth
- **Herbivore**: Above the plane of the molars
- **Omnivore**: On same plane as molar teeth

- **Human**: Above the plane of the molars

Jaw Motion

- **Carnivore**: Shearing; minimal side-to-side motion
- **Herbivore**: No shear; good side-to-side, front-to-back
- **Omnivore**: Shearing; minimal side-to-side
- **Human**: No shear; good side-to-side, front-to-back

Major Jaw Muscles

- **Carnivore**: Temporalis
- **Herbivore**: Masseter and pterygoids
- **Omnivore**: Temporalis
- **Human**: Masseter and pterygoids

Mouth Opening vs. Head Size

- **Carnivore**: Large
- **Herbivore**: Small

- **Omnivore**: Large
- **Human**: Small

Teeth (Incisors)

- **Carnivore**: Short and pointed
- **Herbivore**: Broad, flattened and spade-shaped
- **Omnivore**: Short and pointed
- **Human**: Broad, flattened and spade-shaped

Teeth (Canines)

- **Carnivore**: Long, sharp and curved
- **Herbivore**: Dull and short or long (for defense), or none
- **Omnivore**: Long, sharp and curved
- **Human**: Short and blunted

Teeth (Molars)

- **Carnivore**: Sharp, jagged and blade shaped

- **Herbivore**: Flattened with cusps vs. complex surface
- **Omnivore**: Sharp blades and/or flattened
- **Human**: Flattened with nodular cusps

Chewing

- **Carnivore**: None; swallows food whole
- **Herbivore**: Extensive chewing necessary
- **Omnivore**: Swallows food whole and/or simple crushing
- **Human**: Extensive chewing necessary

Intestinal tract length

The intestinal tracts of carnivorous animals are as many as three to six times their body lengths. The intestinal tracts of herbivores, however, are significantly longer, at 10–12 times longer than their body length. Where do you think human beings fit in? If you guessed herbivores, you're right: human beings actually have the exact same intestinal tract vs. body length ratio as herbivores.

Stomach acidity

A carnivore's stomach is 20x more acidic than an herbivore's stomach. And human beings have the same stomach acidity as an herbivore.

- **Carnivore**: Less than or equal to pH 1 with food in stomach
- **Herbivore**: pH 4 to 5 with food in stomach
- **Omnivore**: Less than or equal to pH 1 with food in stomach
- **Human**: pH 4 to 5 with food in stomach

With this in mind, we can see that a lion can completely digest the flesh, and the process will take him no longer then four to six hours (i.e., the length of time for the meat to enter through the mouth, pass through the digestive system, and exit). Also, as the stomach acidity is much higher in a tiger's stomach that of a human's stomach, it doesn't have a problem with intestinal parasites that live in the flesh, beacause they all get killed with stomach acid. A carnivore can eat rotting, bacteria-ridden flesh completely raw without getting sick. They have stomach acids that can kill the harmful stuff and allow them to digest the rest without puking their guts up. On the contrary, humans must cook their meats.

Have you ever tried to eat roadkill? Or a freshly dead chicken, completely raw? Give it a shot and let me know how it works out for you. E. Coli bacteria, salmonella, campylobacter, trichina worms, parasites, or other pathogens would not survive in the stomach of a carnivore such as a lion. Humans have a much lower stomach acidity, which means if we ingested parasites (along with the dead flesh) they will surely become new "friends" in our intestines and breed into colonies. In addition to that, it takes 24–48 hours (in a congested system it might even take up to four days) for the meat to go through a human'sentire digestive system.

This gives the larvae enough time to develop into parasites and find "a new home" in our gut.

About 99% of people who eat animal products have some kind of worm or parasite, yet they never even question or suspect it. If they don't see them in their stool, they think they don't have them; however, that is a really deceptive point of view.

As a matter of fact, I read an article about a bodybuilder who was 100% healthy and had all the tests, including stool tests done. He was declared "clean" by the doctor's and was very happy. However, one day he got sick and couldn't understand why he had a bloated stomach and severe abdominal pain. When he arrived to the emergency department of the hospital, he ended up going into surgery. The doctors pulled out dozens of ringworms from his gut. He was in shock, as he had never seen them in his stool, nor were the "wonderful" medical tests able to identify this problem.

If we have some rotten putrefying flesh stuck all over our intestinal walls (which takes years and years of eating meat to build this up), then we have to have "friends" to help us clean up all this mess. In this situation, the worms— and all the other kinds of parasites that are invisible to the human eye—are our true friends. However, they also leave waste matter in our intestines, and that is really toxic to us. So, it is best to clean up our intestines and get rid of all this accumulated buildup and mucus. By doing this, we will automatically get rid of our "friends." If they don't have what they eat, they either exit or die.

Stomach Capacity

- **Carnivore**: 60% to 70% of total volume of digestive tract
- **Herbivore**: Less than 30% of total volume of digestive tract
- **Omnivore**: 60% to 70% of total volume of digestive tract
- **Human**: 21% to 27% of total volume of digestive tract

Liver

- **Carnivore**: Can detoxify vitamin A
- **Herbivore**: Cannot detoxify vitamin A
- **Omnivore**: Can detoxify vitamin A
- **Human**: Cannot detoxify vitamin A

Animal flesh is an incredibly complex kind of protein, and needs quite a bit of uric acid in order for that protein to be processed and digested. Our body releases uric acid as needed to break proteins into amino acids. But uric acid is actually toxic, and needs to be flushed out of the body as soon as it is no longer needed (uric acid also contributes to the aging process). Flushing out uric acid is the liver's job—which means that a carnivore's liver must be able to cleanse out as much as 10 times more uric acid than herbivores or omnivores.

Kidneys

- **Carnivore**: Extremely concentrated urine

- **Herbivore**: Moderately concentrated urine
- **Omnivore**: Extremely concentrated urine
- **Human**: Moderately concentrated urine

Saliva

Carnivores have acidic saliva. Herbivores have alkaline salivia, which is helpful in plant food digestion. Guess what kind of saliva humans have? (If you guess alkaline, you're starting to catch on.)

- **Carnivore**: No digestive enzymes
- **Herbivore**: Carbohydrate-digesting enzymes
- **Omnivore**: No digestive enzymes
- **Human**: Carbohydrate-digesting enzymes

Shape of intestines

Carnivore bowels are smooth and don't have any ridges, so that the bowels function similar to a pipe. This lets meat pass through the pipe efficiently and quickly, avoiding any potential buildup of rotting meat. Herbivore bowels, on the other hand, have bumps and ridges alongside their walls that act more like miniature pockets. This allows plant food to pass through slowly and gives the opportunity to absorb more nutrients. The bowels of human beings share the same traits as the bowels of herbivores.

Fiber

Because their digestive tracts are short and smooth, fiber is not a necessity for carnivores. Herbivores need fiber to ensure that food is properly moved through their longer, bumpier digestive tract to ensure that buildups do not occur. Human beings need fiber, putting us in the same category of herbivores once again.

Cholesterol

Carnivores do not need to worry about cholesterol. In fact, they can easily ingest a high-cholesterol diet without experiencing any of the negative side effects. Humans, of course, are another story. Cholesterol absorption is all about the average body temperature. For example, a lion will typically have a body temperature between 100.5 to 102.5 degrees Fahrenheit. A human being has an average body temperature of 97.9, which is significantly lower.

A lion's higher body temperature helps him keep the cholesterol in liquid form and it can pass through the system without any harm. Humans, due to lower body temperature (and blood temperature), have to pay the price for consuming dead animal flesh. Cholesterol is not liquid in a human body, which means it sets in on the walls of arteries and builds up wherever it can in the human system (also, it is the cause of formation of gallstones). In addition to that, humans have zero dietary need for cholesterol because our bodies manufacture all we need. Cholesterol is only found in animal foods, never in plant foods. A plant-based diet is, by definition, a cholesterol-free diet.

Claws and teeth

Carnivores have claws, sharp front teeth capable of subduing prey, and no flat molars for chewing. Herbivores have no claws or sharp front teeth capable of subduing prey, but they do have flat molars for chewing. Humans have the same characteristics as herbivores.

Based on all the above-mentioned facts, it's hard to come to any different conclusion. Most likely we, humans, are meant to consume a plant-based diet.

The myth about calories

What is a calorie? A scientific calorie is a measurement that reflects the amount of energy produced. When measuring calories in food, a scientist calculates the expected output of energy, or how much energy the food will produce for the person consuming it. A dietary calorie is a unit called a kilocalorie, which is equal to 1,000 scientific calories. A dietary calorie, or kilocalorie, is the amount of energy needed to raise the temperature of 1 kilogram of water by 1 degree Celsius.

The original method used to determine the number of kilocalories in a given food directly measured the energy it produced. The food is placed in a bomb calorimeter (which is a sealed container surrounded by water). The food is burned away completely and the resulting rise in water temperature is measured.

The question is: why does no one ever discuss the digestibility of the consumed food? Doesn't a piece of wood have a caloric value too, since it can be burned? If I were to eat wood, wouldn't most of it pass through my body, undigested? All dietary discussions seem to assume that all calories consumed are digested.

To be even more blunt, everyone seems to assume that the caloric content of our fecal output is nil. Is this even true? What if I start a diet comprised entirely of processed foods that are very high in all sorts of chemicals, preservatives, and other toxic matter, including absorption inhibitors (like in soy products)? Or if I start chasing all my Big Macs (if I did eat them) with a dose of laxative? Also, I know for a fact that if I eat 3,000 calories of carrots, I will be losing weight (provided I was on the Standard American Diet prior to that). On the other hand, if I eat 3,000 calories of burgers, I would gain weight and will be extremely obese in a short period of time.

Why does no one question that 3,000 calories of carrots are not equivalent of 3,000 calories of burgers? If carrots are not equal to burgers (provided that the same amount of calories are consumed), then why rely on something that doesn't make sense in the first place?

How can one assume that every person's absorption of foods is the same? For example, if a person has very congested intestines with a lot of plaque hanging on the walls (it usually reaches one inch thick over the decades of buildup on American diet), his/her absorption of food would be roughly 5%. Compare it to a person who has done extensive fasting and cleansing, was on a fruitarian diet for years that melted all that "goo" off the intestinal walls, and has clean intestines. This person's absorption of food would be around 90% or higher. So, the person that has very low percentage of absorption (with congested system) would need to eat 10 times more than the person with a higher absorption in order to receive equal amount of nutrients due to the differences in absorption. How can calories come into account at all?

Clearly, if the first and second person would eat the same amount of calories of the same product, it would affect them differently. If they both ate 3,000 calories of carrots, the first person (with a congested system) would constantly feel hungry and not satisfied, and he/she will start losing weight, clearing his/her system through detoxing. The second person would feel uncomfortable from food overload, and possibly will put on weight from 3,000 calories of the same carrots (especially if they were a fruitarian for years on water-rich fruits).

Also, if the person has heavy metal toxicities (which in most cases the person doesn't even suspect, or is aware of), his/her absorption of certain elements could be 0% no matter how much they consume the needed product. It will all be for nothing until he/she detoxes his/her heavy metal toxicities, because the receptors that are supposed to receive those nutrients are plugged with heavy metals. They act as "a cork in a bottle" and won't allow anything else to reach those receptors.

As you can see from my illustration of examples and the factual support of absurdity of the idea of calories, you can just dismiss the idea of ever counting calories, and make choices based on how toxic or how healing the foods in your diet are.

About blood-type diet

In his original book published in 1997 titled *Eat Right for Your Type*, Dr. D'Adamo asserted a few theories about the evolution of the blood types as well as possible adaptive benefits of the blood type specialization. It turns out that he got these completely wrong. Recent academic studies poke gaping holes in D'Adamo's early evolutionary work. Critics love to harp on the mistakes published in the 1997 book. These mistakes include wrong years for when blood types were first developed, broad speculation about caveman diets, and overall lack of environmental data.

I strongly disagree with the whole concept of a blood type approach. There were a lot of studies conducted proving that people with cancer benefit and can be cured on a raw food diet. However, if a cancer patient keeps eating meat and dairy because of his/her "blood type," then this person dies shortly. My question is: why doesn't the person who keeps eating meat and dairy recover from having cancer (provided it's meant to be the best choice based on their blood type)? Why does the same person get better on a raw vegan diet?

I have all the answers in later chapters where I individually discuss each type of food and how it affects you. There are different people with different blood types that have cancer, yet only the ones that take actions in their own hands, change their lifestyle, and start eating raw fresh vegan foods are able to heal themselves.

I would like to bring to light a comparison of a similar species: monkeys. Do you think that each monkey with a different blood type needs a different diet? Does one monkey need meat and milk, while another needs pizzas, and another needs greens and bananas? I think that this whole idea about blood type is just wrong, because it is confusing people that are trying to find the truth about how to eat properly. I personally tried that blood type diet in my 20s and got severely sick (bloated, stomach cramps, severe constipation, headaches, weakness) within the first three days of trials. What they suggested for my blood type got me sick, not better. I also tried the Atkins diet as well and after three days on that, I had to be in bed for a week recovering from sickness caused by consumption of meats, cheese, and other "goodies" that was suggested by that diet.

In the end, it is an interesting approach of thinking that some humans are naturally born carnivores (based on a blood type); however, in the previous chapter, it is clearly depicted that we are all meant to live on a plant-based diet as suggested by our anatomical structure and system-wide physiological processes.

What are parasites and do we need to kill them?

I recently came across a website written by Thomas Corriher, where all the main aspects of information were summarized in a very nice overview: "Parasites have far surpassed epidemic levels in the United States, with most sources estimating that a massive 85% of Americans have parasitic infections."

Unfortunately, most conventional doctors are not trained in the treatment of parasites. It is only when parasites are visually seen that American doctors will suspect them, but by that time it is already too late. There are many symptoms of parasites that people already display in daily life, believing that these are completely normal. While sickness has become normal in the modern lifestyle, it does not have to be. The amount of damage that can be caused by parasites is limitless, because many are small enough to travel anywhere in the body through the bloodstream. They survive by robbing the body of its nutrients.

Identifying the Different Parasites

- **Roundworms** – These worms live in the stomach and intestines, entering through contaminated or undercooked food. Manure is used in farming, so make sure that you wash all of your produce and wash your hands after interacting with your pets (or their feces).

- **Heartworms** – Heartworms are very rarely found in humans. When they are found (again, only in a few cases has this happened), they tend to show up as one worm in the lung. They cannot be spread from one animal to another (or from one human to another), but they can be carried by mosquitoes.

- **Tapeworms** – These enter the body through beef, fish, or pork that has been undercooked. Tapeworms set up shop in your lower intestinal tract. To avoid tapeworms, you should wear gloves and ensure that you are thoroughly washing your hands after touching unprepared meat.

- **Pinworms** – Pinworms look like tiny, white worms and they live in the lungs and within intestinal tracts. At night, they come out and lay eggs near the anus. Once the eggs hatch, the new worms re-enter through the anus. Scratching while eggs are present means that those pinworm eggs can be transferred from underneath the fingernails to another surface or another person. People may even be able to inhale them, as they are incredibly small and lightweight (perhaps smoking does have a benefit, after all).

- **Hookworms and Threadworms** – These types of parasites live in contaminated drinking water, but they can also enter the body through the soles of the feet. Hookworms and threadworms are both very small, and can pass through the feet even if there are no open cuts or wounds. You should always have shoes on your feet when you are walking around outside. What's unique about hookworms and threadworms is that they can live for years, and have a 10-year incubation period.

- **Flukes** – There are hundreds of varieties of flukes, all in different shapes and forms and colors. They can be in the intestines as well as in your liver, eating holes in its flesh. An average person carries at least five different varieties of flukes, yet has no idea about their existence.

Symptoms of Parasite Infection:

- Intestinal cramping
- Difficulty in sleeping
- Loss of appetite
- Anemia
- Indigestion, bloating

- Chronic, unexplained nausea, often accompanied by vomiting
- Multiple food allergies
- Difficulty maintaining a healthy weight (over or underweight)
- Dizziness
- Palpitations
- Foul-smelling gas
- Fatigue and weakness
- Itching on the soles of the feet, often accompanied by a rash
- Wheezing and coughing, followed by vomiting, stomach pain and bloating
- Coughing blood (severe cases)
- Facial swelling around the eyes
- Itching around the anus, especially at night

Treatment Options:

If you go to the doctor and they diagnose you with parasites, you will get a prescription for a pharmaceutical. Keep in mind, however, that a pharmaceutical is always going to be a toxic substance; after all, it's the toxicity that kills the parasites. Temporary lymph node swelling, and swelling of the hands and feet are common side effects of anti-parasite drugs. You may also experience more serious side effects such as convulsions, difficulty cooordinating movements, or vision impairment.

Treating parasites can be done on your own, without going to the doctor, by using natural-based substances. Here are some of the most common natural ways to get rid of a parasite:

- Garlic
- Black walnut hulls
- Thyme leaf and seed
- Wormwood
- Marshmallow root
- Pumpkin seeds, or pumpkin seed oil capsules
- Neem (Note: Neem is not recommended for pregnant women or for those who are planning on becoming pregnant.)
- Common cloves

Wormwood and black walnut hulls are known to kill adult worms, and cloves can kill worm eggs. Some people use wormwood, black walnut hulls, and cloves together as a trio for treating parasites. The recommended doses are 500 mg. of wormwood and black walnut hulls, and 1/2 teaspoon of cloves. Take these three for about 30 days. All other herbs mentioned are used in addition to these core protocols. (I personally know people who have been taking these herbs for six to eight months to battle their parasitic infections.)

When parasites die, there are toxins released through their excrement and rotting bodies. Wormlike parasites are the most common, and when they are under attack, they will dig deeper into the intestines in an attempt to escape. And even once the parasites are dead, the body will still need to flush them out.

This can cause more pain and more cramps, making you feel sicker instead of better. You can also expect to feel fatigued and groggy—but these are all signs that the treatment is working and that your body is in the cleansing process. Normal bowel movements should commence, and you should be sure to eat a healthy diet to keep your immune system as strong as possible.

My personal opinion is that if you make it so that you cannot be a host for parasites, you will never have to worry about an infection. This means that if your body is detoxed and cleaned well (i.e., all gallstones gone, all the intestines are free from all that buildup of stone fecal matter that was stuck in your intestinal folds that was created over the decades) from most of the toxins and these toxins, including heavy metals, are released from all the connective tissue, joints, muscles, and other cells, there is nothing for parasites to eat or live off. Arnold Ehret, a German naturopath and educator, proved that there cannot be any disease, virus, or parasite that would want to stay in your body if it's clean. It will either die or pass through.

He even proved it with malaria, by putting himself in the most dangerous places where there was an epidemic and intently exposing himself to it, proving the fact that he just can't "catch" it or have it in his healthy body. Also, if you do all the "conventional" harsh medical treatments and get rid of the parasites, you will still get them back within a period of six months through the larva or parasites that have contaminated your foods, water, contact with others, the gym, etc. In most cases, when treating parasites, people wipe out 90% of parasites from their body and feel a relief, not knowing that it's just a short break. By the time they realize what happened, within six months the colonies of their parasites grew back to where they initially started from.

The most important part of this whole story is that you do not want to be a host for parasites. That could be achieved by cleaning up your body and eliminating the parasites permanently with no option for them to return.

Carnivores have all sorts of worms that help the host to decompose all the dead tissue; they are in a sense "little friends" that help to deal with all that garbage that people put and create in their guts and intestines. It is important to bear in mind that these parasites excrete very toxic waste that damages the human system. In addition, parasites will influence what people put in their gut: thus, people have cravings of processed foods full of sugars that would support the life of those parasites, despite being damaging to the host (the human body). Some people complain about the lack of their willpower, but if they would simply get rid of parasites, they will stop having cravings all together—which would be an incredible relief.

I will talk about dry fasting in the later chapters. I believe it is the most potent way to get rid of the parasites. They die from dehydration naturally, without any damage to the body. If you can dry fast (go without food or water) seven to 10 days or at least 72 hours, all your parasites will eventually die. I will describe the needed safety measures and efficiency of this method in a later chapter. Also, dry fasting literally saved my life, as it is very effective in getting rid of toxins. I did a lot of dry fasting. After each dry fast I did, I felt a tremendous improvement with my allergies and was able to eat things that I couldn't before due to my severe reactions. My health was gradually improving, and after each time of dry fasting, I would get a noticeable improvement of my overall well-being that brought me closer to my goal of having infinite health.

What is GMO, and why is it

bad for us?

A GMO (genetically modified organism) is the result of a laboratory process of taking genes from one species and inserting them into another in an attempt to obtain the desired traits or characteristics from both the species. They are also known as transgenic organisms. This process may be called either Genetic Engineering (GE) or Genetic Modification (GM), but no matter which term is used, they are one and the same.

The techniques used to transfer genes have a very low success rate, so the genetic engineers attach "marker genes" that are resistant to antibiotics to help them to find out which cells have taken up the new DNA. These marker genes are resistant to antibiotics that are commonly used in human and veterinary medicine. Some scientists believe that eating GE food containing these marker genes could encourage gut bacteria to develop antibiotic resistance.

The American Academy of Environmental Medicine (AAEM) cites animal studies showing organ damage, gastrointestinal and immune system disorders, accelerated aging, and infertility. And there are human studies that demonstrate GMOs leaving material behind that may cause long-term issues. For example, soy that has been genetically modified could transfer genes into DNA of the "good" bacteria in our bodies. Toxic insecticides in genetically modified corn has been found within the bloodstreams of pregnant women (and even in the blood of unborn fetuses).

There has been a substantial increase in health issues following the introduction of genetically modified organisms in the late 1990s. In nine years' time, the number of Americans with at least three chronic illnesses increased from 7% to 13%; food allergies have exploded; and we are seeing digestive issues, reproductive challenges, and autism all increasing in frequency.

The majority of GMO crops are meant to be tolerant to weed killers (herbicides). "Roundup Ready" crops are sold by Monsanto, and these are all meant to be impervious to Roundup herbicide. GMO crops received an additional 383 million pounds of herbicide between the years of 1996 and 2008. Unfortunately, the widespread use of Roundup creates weeds that are completely resistant to herbicide, which causes farmers to create more advanced herbicides to protect their crops. It's a deadly cycle that not only creates environmental damage, but it also causes toxic residue on GMO crops. Herbicides (and Roundup in particular) are commonly associated with hormonal disruption, cancer, birth defects, and sterility.

There are plenty of side effects that come as a result of GMOs. The whole idea of creating genetically modified crops means that you are combining genes from one species with the genes of another (and often completely unrelated) species. That makes it difficult to predict what type of side effects may be caused, as that genetic mixup has little to no precedent. By relying heavily on GMOs, we may be inadvertently introducing never-before-seen allergens, toxins, and carcinogens.

So where did GMOs begin, and how did they gain FDA approval? Well, the Flavr Savr tomato was the first GMO product that was submitted to the FDA for review and approval. Studies showed that there were toxins present in the genetically modified tomato. In a lab rat study, seven out of 20 subjects were shown to have stomach lesions after eating the Flavr Savr. Arpad Pusztai, Ph.D., is one of the leading global experts in assessing the safety of GMOs. He says that the stomach lesions displayed after eating the genetically modified tomatoes "could lead to life-endangering hemorrhage, particularly in the elderly who use aspirin to prevent [blood clots]." He concluded that the digestive tract (as the primary and largest point of contact with food) should be the first point of analysis when looking at the risk of GMOs.

Of course, the impact of the Flavr Savr tomato on the intestines was never studied by the FDA.

Outside of the FDA, there have been other studies that focused on analyzing the effect of GMOs on the intestines. For example, a study was conducted where mice were given potatoes that contained an extra gene, a bacteria that created Bt-toxin (an insecticide). After looking at the lower section of the small intestine, scientists discovered cells that had been damaged, as well as cells that were displaying abnormal or increased cell growth. Similar results were seen with rats that were fed GMO potatoes that were engineered with a different kind of pesticide. The issue here is that rapid cell growth is a significant concern whenever it is observed, as it can open the door to cancer development.

Because the liver is the primary detoxifier, analyzing liver health is a good way to determine the presecne of toxins. In the case of the rats that were fed genetically modified potatoes, their lives were much smaller and even somewhat atrophied. Rats that consumed corn (Bt-toxin) contracted lesions on their livers. Rabbits that ate genetically modified soy showed both increased metabolic activity and changes to enzyme production within the liver. Rats that ate canola that was "Roundup Ready" had livers that were 12%–16% heavier, which could potentially be from inflammation or a type of disease. Mice that ate soybeans that were "Roundup Ready" had livers with disrupted gene structure and functional adjustments. Once the diet was changed to foods that were not genetically modified, many issues went away, leading us to believe that the genetically modified crops were the source of liver issues.

There are other studies that have displayed increased death rates in animals that were fed GMOs. For example, during the Flavr Savr tomato study, there were seven rats that perished after two weeks. Chickens that consumed GMO corn were dying two times faster than chickens that ate regular corn. The most important note about this all is that, in the case of both studies, these deaths were briefly mentioned and then set aside (without any sort of additional explanation or investigation).

Within the pancreas of mice that were fed "Roundup Ready" soy, the organ showed many changes and was creating fewer digestive enzymes than in the control group of mice. For rats, their pancreas was larger than normal. Kidney functions in various animals were altered significantly, including inflammation, changed enzyme produciton, lesions, and increased toxicity. Mice that ate genetically modified soy had interrupted enzyme production, while rats showed slower brain growth in rats.

In both mice and rats that were fed Roundup Ready soybeans, their testicles showed dramatic changes. The rats showed organs that had turned from pink into dark blue. Young sperm cells in mice were changed as a result of Roundup Ready soybeans. And in the embryos of mice that were fed soy, scientists observed temporary alterations in genetic function when compared to adult mice that ate non-GM soy.

Further dramatic results were discovered by a leading scientist at the Russian National Academy of sciences. Female rats were fed GM soy, starting from two weeks before they mated. According to the Arizona Center for Advanced Medicine, in the course of three different experiments, more than 50% of the offspring died from the group that was fed GMO soy. Compare this to only 10% from the group that ate non-GMO soy and approximately 8% from the control group that did not eat soy at all. As reported by Irina Ermakova, "High pup mortality was a characteristic of every litter from mothers that were fed the GM soy flour." Even the average size and weight of the GM-fed offspring was reported to be significantly smaller. Initial studies showed that offspring of rats that were fed GMO soy were unable to reproduce.

Once the three trials were complete, the rat food supplier at the Russian lab started to incorporate GM soy. That meant that all rats at

the laboratory were now consuming GM soy,
eliminating the possibility of having a control
group for any further trials. Unfortunately,
follow-up experiments were cancelled. As
reported by the Arizona Center for Advanced
Medicine, two months into a diet of genetically
modified soy, however, the lab rats were
suffering from an extremely high infant
mortality rate, at more than 55%.

Approximately 24 farmers said that
feeding their pigs certain kinds of genetically
modified corn (Bt corn) resulted in thousands
of pigs experiencing reproductive issues. These
complications ranged from sterility to false
pregnancies and even births that weren't births
at all (sacs of water). Cows and bulls have also
encountered sterility issues from Bt corn, while
deaths of chickens, horses, cows, and water
buffaloes have also been connected to various
strains of genetically modified corn.

From 2006 to 2007, Indian shepherds
allowed sheep to graze on genetically modified
cotton plans. They found that, in a week or less,
one in four sheep died. In 2006, there were as

many as 10,000 sheep deaths, a number which increased the next year. The sheep showed significant intenstinal and liver irritation, along with black patches and enlarged bile ducts. The Arizona Center for Advanced Medicine reports that, according to investigators, evidence "strongly suggests that the sheep mortality was due to a toxin... most probably Bt-toxin."

What does this tell us? Almost every single independent study focusing on animals eating GM foods demonstrates serious negative effects—but the biotech industry has done a superb job at keeping these studies suppressed. They don't want us to know that GMOs are harmful. In fact, the studies discussed in the previous paragraphs were not able to be peer-reviewed or published. Lawsuits are the only reason they are available in any form today. And many scientists and researchers who have been looking into complications from genetically modified foods have been silenced in other ways: they have been fired, demoted, or threatened. Despite all of this, we are still being fed the narrative that genetically modified crops are just as safe as natural crops.

So what kinds of crops are being genetically modified in the US? In 2014, Onset Worldwide listed tthe GMO landscape as the following:

- Soy (94%)
- Cotton (90%)
- Sugar beets (95%)
- Corn (88%)
- Hawaiin papaya (50+%)
- Zucchini and yellow squash (over 24,000 acres)

GMOs don't stop at vegetables and fruits, either. Products that come from genetically modified crops can be equally as harmful. This includes oils, cornstarch, corn syrup, soy protein, and more. And don't forget about all of the animals that eat genetically modified crops (which applies to most of the genetically modified corn and soy in the US). Milk, cheese, and other dairy products may be contaminated by cows injected with genetically modified hormones. Even honey may have been contaminated by bee pollen with a genetically modified source. There are also plenty of items outside of your kitchen pantry that could have GMOs in them, such as soaps, detergents, cosmetics, shampoo and conditioner, and even vitamins and supplements.

It seems to me that not many people actually understand what GM foods could do to human health, even though they have heard about them. I personally encountered this situation while getting my fruits at the grocery store. As I was putting some apples in my cart, an elderly lady asked me if I liked corn (as she was putting it in her grocery bag). I told her that I did like corn, but I would never touch it in America because 90% of corn in America is GMO, unfortunately. She asked me, "What does GMO mean?" I tried to explain to her, but she shook her head and said, "I wish I didn't ask you," as she kept putting more corn in her basket.

What can I say? Some people believe whatever they want to believe, which is the importance of having a good meal in the evening, including comfort foods that you are used to eating since childhood. Even if it's GMO corn, it's okay.

People have a tendency to believe that huge corporations will put the well-being of people over their profit. It is hard for them to accept that some veggies and even fruits are GMO and that they are not the same as non-GMO fruits and veggies. In the end, food looks the same and tastes the same; therefore, it must be harmless, because it doesn't kill us instantly (it does in long run, but no one is paying attention).

It is the same story with organic and non-organic items as well. People know that organic foods are good and that non-organic foods are not so good, but they don't realize why. They don't really know that non-organic foods are more likely to be GMO as well, and that they are heavily sprayed with pesticides that are detrimental to our health.

I will never forget the story about one girl who was supposedly allergic to carrots. One day, she ate an organic carrot and was totally fine. When she tried going back to non-organic carrots, she had the same symptoms of "allergies." Apparently, she had a reaction to pesticides in the non-organic carrots.

Since I learned all this, I got really careful about what I was putting in my basket at the grocery store. Even though I was considering buying organic zucchini sometimes, I just couldn't shake off that feeling that zucchini might be GMO as well (considering the statistics in the US). Also, grocery store workers don't really care if a pile of non-organic veggies gets confused with organic, and non-organic items end up in organic section (I have heard of such accidents that happened to my friend more than once when he worked his shift at Whole Foods, of all places). Therefore, I try to avoid all the big-production GMO food groups that I mentioned above altogether. I try to avoid potatoes, zucchini, squashes, and other items that would be more likely GMOs. I also try to get heirloom foods and foods from farmer's markets in order to avoid all that toxic non-organic and GMO stuff.

As they say, "Ignorance is bliss." Sometimes I wonder how wonderful it would be not to know what I do. Then, I would be careless about where and what to eat. I would have been able to enjoy any and every type of food under the sun (including cooked and animal products, as well as all fast food chain restaurants that are very toxic). I would have never even have considered the possibility of deterioration of my health being the direct result of what I was eating. I would have been eaily able to enjoy that wide variety of flavors and indulge in different dishes—but I would be paying a *very* high price with my health, just like every ignorant human being does.

On the other hand, I am thankful that I took my time to research every detail about nutrition and foods, where they come from, and how they affect our bodies. I am grateful that I had the opportunity to take matters of my health in my own hands and not depend on anyone else's opinion—you can't go against facts.

We are what we eat, but doctors in our society do not believe it. Genetically modified food is not the only culprit in the declining overall health of Americans. They will "cure" you to death with pills, "therapies," and surgeries. Doctors are the same victims of our society. Just like us, they are programmed with false information and have no idea about the truth. As a matter of fact, they don't even take one class about nutrition throughout their studies to be a doctor. Only a few would take it upon themselves to go on a journey to research the truth and find it.

Is dairy bad for the human system and why?

In his book, *Herbal Health Care*, John R. Christopher, N.D., M.H., writes: "There is a tremendous difference between human babies and baby calves and a corresponding difference between the milk intended to nourish human babies and the milk intended to nourish baby calves." It takes about 180 days for a human infant to double its birth weight, and human milk consists of 5% to 7% protein. It takes only 45 days for a calf to double its birth weight, and cow's milk is 15% protein. This protein in cow's milk is of a different composition than that of human milk and is poorly assimilated in the human body. The primary type of protein in cow's milk is casein. According to Dr. Christopher, there is up to 20 times more casein in cow's milk than in human milk, which makes the nutrients in cow's milk difficult (if not impossible) for humans to assimilate.

I would like to stress upon the situation in the US (I am not sure if it's the same in Europe). Processed or raw milk has traces of antibiotics and Bovine Growth hormone in it. Without Bovine Growth hormone, the farmers would be out of business. It is a tough competition, and farmers have to find cheap ways to increase milk production. Bovine Growth Hormone is a genetically engineered hormone created by Monsanto. There has been controversy across the nation over the use of Bovine Growth Hormone, which is referred to as either rBGH or rBST. Farmers who use Bovine Growth Hormone will inject cows with this bioengineered hormone every two weeks to stimulate increased milk production. Although this hormone is similar (certainly not identical) to the naturally produced milk-inducing hormones, there are plenty of negative side effects for the cows that wouldn't occur otherwise. The penalty for increased milk production is higher levels of pus, leftover antibiotics residues, and the creation of a cancer-accelerating hormone (IGF-1).

As the cows are forced into higher milk production, their bodies are more susceptible to udder infections, a condition called mastitis. Mastitis causes the udders to become inflamed, increasing the amount of pus that is transferred into the milk. The label for Posilac (the brand name for rBGH) even states that this is a known side effect: "Cows injected with Posilac are at an incrased risk for mastitis (visibly abnormal milk) and may have higher somatic cell counts...Cows injected with Posilac may require more therapeutic drug treatment for mastitis and other health problems."

The warning label also mentions other side effects, such as body temperature changes and swelling: "Cows injected with Posilac may have more enlarged hocks and disorders of the foot region. Posilac treatment may reduce hemoglobin and hematocrit values."

Treating mastitis is best done through an antiobiotics regimen, which only increases the traces of antibiotics that are found in the milk jugs we purchase at the grocery store. Those who support the use of rBGH state that milk is an incredibly regulated food when it comes to antibiotic residue (one of the highest regulations overall). According to these sources, each batch of milk is thoroughly tested before packaging to ensure that there are no antibiotics present—and if there are any trace amounts found, the entire batch of milk is destroyed. And this testing occurs at a farm-by-farm level, with each farmer's batch being tested for antibiotics before it is even picked up. Should the presence of antibiotics be found, the farmer would be penalized by being charged for an entire tank of milk.

While the above might seem comforting, it's worth mentioning that only four out of 82 commercially used antibiotics are typically tested for. Compounding the problem is the fact that additional antibiotics that are not legal for use are somehow found our milk. In a widely cited study by The Wall Street Journal (B. Ingersoll, December 1989), a study of the antibiotic residues in milk found that 20% of milk on the marketplace had illegal antibiotics present. In a 1990 study by *Consumer Reports* titled "Biotechnology and Milk: Benefit or Threat?" this number was confirmed (along with the increased rates of udder infections). The Center for Science in the Public Interest found that 38% of milk was contamined by antibiotics that had not been officially approved for use. Despite regulation, it seems as though the economic benefit of having cows produce more milk outweighed the risk in introducing the American public to illegal, untested antibiotics.

When rBGH is present in a cow's body, their blood starts producing another type of homrone, called Insulin-Like Growth Factor-1 (IGF-1). This secondary hormone is what causes an increase in milk production. IGF-1 is a naturally occuring hormone for both cows and humans (it helps boost cell growth in infants, which is why it is a natural component of breastmilk) but the rate of production when introduced to a bioengineered hormone is anything but natural. To put this in perspective, IGF-1 is increased nearly five times higher with the use of rBGH. Humans already create IGF-1 hormones naturally, but it is typically bound to a protein and has a much more muted effect than what we see in milk (i.e., when IGF-1 is not bound to a protein).

As cow's milk is introduced into an adult's diet, it becomes an accelerant for cancer. IGF-1 isn't digested, so it stays biologically active within our body, promoting cellular division. When cells divide, they only stop dividing due to hormonal and genetic signals, called "programmed cell death." If "programmed cell death" is interrupted and cells are enabled to multiply unchecked, their growth grows out of of control—in other words, cancer occurs. IGF-1 has been connected with colon, breast, and prostate cancers.

Both Monsanto and the FDA have joined forces to pressure any markets that attempt to label milk and dairy products as "rBGH-free." In some cases, they have even filed lawsuits to keep the label from appearing. Both corporations have lied about testing capabilities for rBGH in milk; according to the Energy Justice Network: "Monsanto has tried to block publication of a research from British scientists on rBGH showing the hormone's link to increased somatic cell (pus and bacteria) counts in milk as a result of mastitis."

Further reports from the Energy Justice Network are just as dire, if not more so. Consider this excerpt from an article titled "Bovine Growth Hormone: Milk does nobody good":

"Monsanto admitted to receiving 95 reports in the first six months of sales from farmers with problems. Thirty-six cows treated with the drug died and 14 farmers have reported problems with mastitis. Monsanto did not report the case of a farmer in Florida who lost nine cows and stated that another 15% of his herd needed to be culled (killed). His milk was rejected due to high pus content as a result of mastitis. This follows the same pattern as the farmer in New York who lost a quarter of his dairy herd to rBGH and the multiple reports from farmers who lost small numbers of cows shortly after introduction of rBGH, due to things like internal hemorrhaging."

Monsanto is the only one who is benefitting from rBGH. Even the FDA has said that consumers see no benefit from the genetically engineered hormone. Energy Justice Network warns that the Consumers Union has predicted that rBGH "will cost the taxpayer an additional $200 million in surplus milk that the government (your taxes) will buy up to keep the milk prices stable. This is in a nation where we've spent an average of $2.1 billion each year from 1980 to 1985 buying surplus milk."

From 1986 to 1987, farmers were paid by the government to slaughter cows and halt any dairy farming for a five-year period. This voluntary program had 14,000 participants, resulting in the deaths of more than 1.5 million dairy cows. Though we continue to have an excess of milk supplies (and cows are already under undue stress to continuously produce more milk), Monstanto continues to profit from rBGH, a bioengineered hormone that amounts to little more than a widespread, low-cost social experiment on their part. Whether milk is raw or processed, it already has destructive components in it, including Bovine Growth Hormone, antibiotics, and IGF-1.

Let's pretend that there are none of the above mentioned components in milk: would it still be good for the human body, or would it be toxic?

Many heavily researched books and articles have demonstrated that processed cow's milk does not have health benefits for human consumption. On the other side of the spectrum, it has actually been associated with a number of physiological issues. These include: acne, arthritis, sinusitis, iron deficiency, anemia, osteoporosis, colic, gastrointestinal bleeding, allergies, heart disease, skin rashes, diarrhea, diabetes, and autoimmune disease. It's even possible that processed cow's milk has connections to multiple sclerosis, lung cancer, and non-Hodgkin's lymphoma.

Milk and dairy both promote acid and mucus production in the body, making it easier for children and adults alike to contract flus and colds more easily.

Raw milk has good bacteria in it, which is why raw milk eventually curdles when sitting at room temperature. In contrast, pasteurized milk eliminates enzymes and decreases overall vitamin content by as much as half. And without any good bacteria or enzymes, pasteurized milk will eventually rot—even if it is not left out at room temperature. And pasteurized milk has been shown to be extremely detrimental in studies: in one study, calves who were fed pasteurized milk died in 60 days or less.

If it's so unhealthy for us, why would we even want to pasteurize milk? First, it makes the shelf life for milk much longer. Unpasteurized milk will last only five days or so, while pasteurized milk can last for weeks. Second, pasteurized milk goes through a sanitation process, meaning that the cleanliness standards for farmers are less strict.

Carl W. Hall and G. Malcom Trout, in their book *Milk Pasteurization*, state: "Pasteurization is an excuse for the sale of 'dirty' milk. Unfortunately, dairies often milk cows with manure heavily coated on the hind legs. The milk suction tubes can easily rub against these filthy areas. The teats are supposed to be carefully wiped off before milking.

In poorly supervised operations, the milker carries a paper towel in the back pocket of his jeans. Sometimes he wipes off the teats, and sometimes he doesn't. So, you end up having pus, feces, mud, and urine in your milk even if it has been heated."

Heat destroys a great number of bacteria in milk (but not all of them) and conceals the evidence of dirt. The toxin from bacteria responsible for diarrhea, the enterotoxin, is largely unaffected by pasteurization. If raw milk is contaminated to a significant degree, you can instantly tell that it is, from the smell and taste. But pasteurized milk may be seriously contaminated with no telltale odor or taste at all.

The milk is devitalized. Pasteurization diminishes vitamin content and destroys vitamin C. Added vitamins and minerals in the milk, at the end of the process, are not bio-available to our body. Our body sees them as non-organic toxic matter. There is no use for any of the added vitamins or minerals; instead, they cause the body harm. There is a very short-lived effect from them in the system, and afterwards, our body tries to "hide" away this inorganic matter in our body tissues, joints, and bones, or encapsulates them in gallstones to protect our system from toxic poison (as our liver can't process all the poison we put in our bodies on daily basis). It's an accumulative effect to health deterioration over the years.

Dr. William Campbell Douglass mentions in *The Milk Book* that heating the milk turns the lactose into beta-lactose, which is far more soluble and therefore more rapidly absorbed into the blood stream. As Dr. Douglass says: "The sudden rise in blood sugar is followed by a fall leading to low blood sugar and hypoglycemia, which induces hunger. The end result is obesity. Pasteurized milk makes you fat, raw milk does not." Obesity has become one of the most common diseases of childhood.

Calcium and other minerals are precipitated and made unavailable by pasteurization. The complete destruction of the enzyme phosphatase is one testing method to determine whether the milk has been adequately pasteurized. This enzyme is essential for the absorption of calcium, but it is completely destroyed in the process of pasteurization. Pasteurization disintegrates salts like calcium, iron and phosphates, causing them to lose their organic quality and making them impossible (or, at best, extremely difficult) to assimilate.

Infants don't develop well on pasteurized milk. Pasteurized milk is more likely to lead to decay in teeth, as it interferes with the proper development of the teeth and creates a predisposition to cavities. As William Campbell Douglass warns in *The Milk Book*: "Remember that your teeth are the window to your body's physical condition. They reflect your general state of health. If your teeth are deteriorating, YOU are deteriorating. Hardening of the arteries and decaying teeth are part of the same degenerative process. The one you can see, cavities, comes early in life. The other, atherosclerosis—heart attack, is not seen and comes later. They are a continuum— one of the main parts of the same degenerative process leading to disease and death. Pasteurized milk is more likely to be constipating. Pasteurization would lead to an increase in infant mortality as it also diminishes resistance to disease (especially in young babies)."

Pasteurization destroys beneficent enzymes, antibodies, and hormones which takes the life out of milk. For example, the enzyme lipase is completely destroyed by the pasteurization process. Lipase aids in the digestion of fats. The complete destruction of lipase is imperative, otherwise the milk becomes rancid. Also, pasteurization destroys the souring bacteria of milk so that instead of souring, milk will normally putrefy if kept-out long enough. Pasteurization kills the bacilli in milk and causes it to decompose when exposed to air (bacterial corpse).

The following excerpt from *The Milk Book* provides an in-depth overview of how pasteurized milk can be so detrimental:

There are serious allergies heat-processed milk has caused among children and adults alike. Pasteurized milk allergy, caused by altering the milk proteins through heating, has caused a major health problem in the United States." "In one investigation detailing the "heat treatment" of milk, it was revealed that not just one simple heating takes place. Milk is heated over again with each process. In clarification, the milk may be heated to 135°F. In the filtering process, the milk is heated again upto about 100°F. In the bactofugation process (method of removing bacteria), the milk is again heated to 170°F. With deaeration a vacuum treatment is used in which the milk is treated in two vacuum chambers, the first at 175°F, the second 100°-152°F.

Bulk storage of milk has led to off-flavor (tainting). Food Engineering Magazine has the answer; "Blanching", which means heating the milk again! These heats may vary according to the system used, but the milk is heated over and over again. It is hard to imagine this milk resembling the original product after all of this steam-cleaning.

The research showed that clarification was necessary to prevent the sedimentation found, even in aseptically produced milk, which was the result of settling out of leucocytes in milk that had been homogenized. The average reader would not know what leucocytes are, so I'll tell you; PUS—that's right, just plain pus. In addition to pasteurization and with the onset of homogenization, a very undesirable situation had developed. The leucocytes (pus) were noted to settle to the bottom of the bottle and make a grayish oil-like sludge. One can't sell milk with a pus layer, and, as almost all milk is now homogenized, something had to be done to get this out, so the clarification process was instituted. The sediment removed by the clarification process is called in the milk trade, slime—and that is PUS.

Another chemical that can be found in the cow's milk is organo-phosphate. Many diaries are now feeding an organo-phosphate to their cattle. This chemical, known as lincophos, ends up in the manure and poisons the larvae of flies.

Why maintain a clean barn when you can just dose your cows with organo-phosphate and let the chemically contaminated manure poison the maggots? This affects the pituitary gland in cows that affects the level and production of hormones (which is in the cow's milk), which leads to diabetes, hypertension, Addison's Disease, acne, and many more dysfunctions. In turn, this abnormal reaction of hormone imbalance of cows reflects on the quality of their milk that is not "normal" by far any longer.

I highly recommend *The Milk Book* by William Campbell Douglass where he addresses the subject of milk in detail (as well as the information mentioned above) starting from milking farms, the process of "cleaning" the milk, to the final stage of how we end up with such poor health conditions if we consume processed milk. He states that "skim or low-fat milk may cause degenerative arthritis, also called calcific arthritis."

Calcification of other tissues such as the pineal gland, arteries, and kidneys are caused by drinking fractionated (skim, non-fat) milk. There is a little gland right in the center of the skull called the pineal gland. This gland is often calcified, even in young people. The pineal gland is extremely important in light physiology and hormonal regulation in humans. Skim milk-fed animals develop testicular atrophy with complete sterility. Male sterility is a major concern in the US today, and the skim milk fast may be a major contribution factor. Millions of people are drinking low-fat milk to avoid weight gain.

Do you know how a farmer fattens his hogs? He feeds them skim milk. You can find more details on all the experiments (there are many of them detailed in *The Milk Book* that were done to prove the point of how treated milk is damaging to our health, and what kind of chemicals are added to the milk to make it last longer). In the United States, patients drinking processed milk had a three-fold higher incidence of heart attacks. In England, the heavy processed milk drinkers had a six-fold increase in heart attacks as compared to the non-milk users.

Another important aspect of milk processing is homogenization. I learned from *The Milk Book*, that:

In the homogenization process, the fat particles of the cream are broken up. This is done by straining the fat through tiny pores under great pressure. The resulting fat particles are so small (one-millionth of a meter) that they stay in suspension. So the cream is evenly distributed throughout the milk.

Homogenizing milk has been linked to the rise in arteriosclerosis (hardening of the arteries) and heart disease. The culprit is an enzyme in milk called xanthine oxidase (XO) that partly survives pasteurization (40 percent). When the cream in milk is in its natural state, the fat globules are too large to go through the intestinal wall and into the bloodstream. Homogenization changes that by straining the fat through tiny pores under great pressure. XO attaches itself to the fat molecules (now reduced in size but increased in amount a hundred times), which are now small enough to get into the bloodstream and do its damage. Scientists have discovered that a significant amount of XO is present in areas of hardened and blocked arteries. XO is not present in human milk. In clean, raw cow's milk, XO is not absorbed by the intestines.

In addition to that, we've also got another problem. You know the Vitamin D that the milk producers have so kindly added to your milk? Firstly, it isn't a vitamin. It's a hormone, like cortisone. Secondly, it is helping XO harden your arteries. Doctors Ross and Oster have discovered that D3, the one they add to pasteurized milk and other processed foods, activates XO. In the presence of testosterone, the male sex hormone, it activates XO even more. So a male, drinking pasteurized, homogenized, Vitamin D milk is really asking for it.

Your bones are a mineral bank for your body storing 99 percent calcium, 85 percent phosphorus and 60 percent magnesium. When mineral levels are low in the blood, osteoclasts break down bone to free up these minerals and deposit them in the blood. Excessive animal protein intake increases the need for calcium to neutralize the acid formed from digesting animal protein.

This indicates that the drinking of processed milk destroys bone in the process of digestion which is the opposite of what the Dairy Farmer's Association of America, the U.S. Department of Agriculture and the Food and Drug Administration has been telling the American public for generations.

Jethro Kloss, author of the internationally recognized and revered herbalist resource guide "Back to Eden" stated in 1939 that, "Cow's milk is unfit for human consumption" and causes the symptoms of "intestinal auto-intoxication."

We all know that cow's milk has calcium in it—no questions about it. But how much of that calcium can our body actually digest and use? Every one of us has been told to drink milk so that we can have strong teeth and strong bones. Interestingly enough, although the US has the highest dairy product consumption across the globe, it also has the highest rates of osteoporosis and bone fractures. According to the January 1988 edition of *The Journal of Clinical Endocrinology and Metabolism*, a study found that calcium excretion and bone loss increases as the amount of animal protein is ingested. Because they have a high sulfur content, animal proteins change the way that the kidneys absorb calcium. Instead of absorbing more calcium, a diet that his rich in meats, eggs, and dairy products actually means that an individual is losing more calcium than they are gaining. These individuals, on average, are excreting approximately 90–100 miligrams of calcium each day.

I also learned from *The Milk Book* about milk substitutes. See the following excerpt for more details:

> You may now purchase, from your neighborhood grocer, pasteurized, homogenized dipotassium and calcium phosphate, with hydrogenated vegetable fat, sodium caseinate, sugar (of course), artificial flavoring (of course), guar gum, "NATURAL color," carrageenan, salt, and all blended with that wonderful food, sodium silicoaluminate. To those of you who are not chemistry professors, that is also known as sand.
>
> One of the biggest get-rich schemes since the Florida land boom and the Dutch tulip craze is the high-powered promotion

now going on for these milk substitutes made from the waste product of cheese production called whey. Business has been so phenomenal that the companies have gone into night shifts according to one promoter. Automated equipment has been installed that will enable them to produce 7,500 pounds a minute. Even America's cows look like lactating mice in comparison.

The dairymen used to throw the whey down the drain, but it clogged the sewers. They tried fermenting it for methane gas production which was unsuccessful as well. Feeding it to the pigs seemed a good idea, but even the pigs didn't like it, so they used it for fertilizer. It's known as "the whey disposal problem."

The general rule seems to be, "When all else fails, feed it to humans." So a Salt Lake City outfit took whey residue, threw in some sugar, coconut oil, a bunch of

GRAS chemicals (stand for Generally Regarded as Safe—I wish that statement "safe" was true...), and five synthetic vitamins, and presto—a product that is "33% to 42% more nutritious then milk!... Pigs and people wouldn't eat whey because it tastes awful. But junk food promoters have proven that the American people will eat anything if you put enough sugar and artificial flavoring in it and call it "natural" and "nutritious."

To increase dietary calcium, consider increasing your consumption of green leafy vegetables such as collards, kale, and spinach. I also found it useful to substitute milk with a much better option, such as almond milk or coconut milk that I make myself to ensure that no preservatives or non-organic chemicals are added in it.

To make almond milk, take a couple of handfuls of raw unpasteurized almonds, and put them in the blender (I use VitaMix) with four cups of water. If you like your milk sweet, add one or two dates. Blend it all together, and then strain through a nut-milk bag. Your milk is ready to be used: it's that simple. It lasts a couple of days in the fridge. Make sure to stir it before using, as it will separate in the fridge.

Coconut milk is much smoother and is, by far, my favorite. Also, coconut milk helps to treat intestinal parasites. To make coconut milk, take one brown mature coconut, crack it open, and strain the water into the sink (I don't use that water, because it doesn't taste sweet). Take the entire meat of the nut (the inside of coconut) and put it in the blender. You can add coconut water from a young coconut (if you want it sweeter), or just four to six cups of regular water (I use Reverse Osmosis water). Blend it all and strain through the nut-milk bag. Your milk is ready. It is by far more tasty than any cow's milk and a much healthier option.

Is cheese good for you? And why is it so addictive?

Cheese was the hardest thing in the world for me to give up. I was a big cheese eater; in fact, I would make my entire dinner out of cheese. My whole family was a huge fan of cheese. And how about pizza? It was my absolute favorite meal.

When I learned about how damaging cheese is to my health, I was determined to give it up. However, it was easier said than done. When I gave it up, I was dreaming about it. Only the knowledge that it caused my allergies, mucus accumulation and buildup in my system, constipation, and high toxicity was holding me back. It took me about a year until the urge to eat cheese fell off by itself, and I was not tormented with the idea of (and the dreams) of eating it again. All efforts paid off in the end, and I now look back at my path of torments and wonder: why was I so attached and addicted to cheese? Not only am I *not* craving that nasty stuff anymore, I am even grossed out by it now. How could someone, in all common sense, want to eat that processed mucus with pus, blood, and feces that smells like dirty socks?

When I quit, I didn't give into my urges to eat cheese: instead, I had an alternative. I was making my own cheese from raw, unpasteurized almonds. I would take almonds and soak them in water for at least six hours (but it's best if they are soaked overnight). The brown skin of an almond contains an enzyme inhibitor. This protects the almond until the right sunlight and moisture levels are reached, allowing it to germinate. Almonds don't release those enzymes until they get enough moisture and sunlight—and without releasing enzymes, you are limiting the amount of nutrients your body can absorb (and making the almonds harder to digest).

Soaking almonds helps remove the nut from its shell and releases enzymes. This is a process that you can use with nearly all nuts and seeds. After I soak my almonds, I peel off the shells (they pop out of that thin brown shell after being soaked very easily under gentle pressure of two fingers). Next, I put them in the blender (Vitamix) and blend one cup of almonds for every half cup of water (it could take more water—the idea is to make it thick, like a sour cream consistency when blended). I open one capsule of probiotics and put them in my blender as well. Once it's blended, you have to put the blended mixture in a nut milk bag, and put it under pressure to strain the remaining water overnight in room temperature.

The following morning, the cheese is done. It will be the same as cream cheese consistency, and you can put any fillers you like in it. For example, you can add a dash of Himalayan Pink salt, you can add finely chopped dill, or parsley, or cilantro, or all of them together. You can add chopped sun-dried tomatoes (soaked for 20 mins), or Italian seasoning. Be creative: it's your cheese, and you can make it any flavor you want.

Cheese is made from milk (see the previous chapter above about milk), so I won't even get into a deep discussion of how detrimental it is to our health. Because cheese is a concentration of milk, you get much more milk and cream in a compressed version of cheese. But have you ever felt like you couldn't give up cheese? Does it sometimes feel like you are addicted to it? In the 1980s, researchers discovered that cheese actually contains small amounts of morphine.

According to Dr. Neal D. Barnum: "In 1981, Eli Hazum and his colleagues at Wellcome Research Laboratories in Research Triangle Park, NC, reported a remarkable discovery. Analyzing samples of cow's milk, they found traces of a chemical that looked very much like morphine. They put it to one chemical test after another. And, finally, they arrived at the conclusion that, in fact, it is morphine. There's not a lot of it and not every sample had detectable levels. But there is indeed some morphine in both cow's milk and human milk. As FreeFromHarm.org reports:

Researchers also discovered the protein casein that breaks into casomorphins when it is digested and also produces opiate effects. In cheese, casein is concentrated, so is the level of casomorphins, so the pleasurable effect is greater. Neal Barnard, MD said, 'Since cheese is processed to express out all the liquid, it's an incredibly concentrated source of casomorphins,you might even call it dairy crack.' (Source: VegetarianTimes.com)

One research paper states, 'Casomorphins are peptides produced from the breakdown of CN and possess opioid activity. The term opioid refers to morphine-like effects which include signs of sedation, tolerance, sleep induction, and depression.' (Source: University of Illinois Extension.)

And another research study conducted in Russia found that a type of casomorphin found in cow milk might impact human infant development negatively, specifically in a manner resembling autism.

To make matters worse, cheese also contains saturated fat and cholesterol, which contribute to heart disease, and formation of gallstones. One ounce of cheese can contain a large amount of saturated fat.

In 2013, in an article titled "You Really Can't Eat Just One, and Here's the Reason" by Scott Mowbray, the *New York Times* reported that Americans now consume about 33 pounds of cheese each year. Limiting cheese and saturated fat intake are easy steps that anyone can take to reduce the chance of heart disease. This is of particular importance for the US, since some have estimated that an unhealthy diet and a lack of exercise could be responsible for anywhere between 300,000 to 500,000 deaths per year (as reported by FreeFromHarm.org). Decreasing cheese intake is easier said than done, since cheese produces opiate-like effects within our brain. It's a constant battle: if you want to regain full health and all of the benefits, you have to go to war with YOURSELF.

The truth about ice cream

When eating ice cream, one doesn't usually think about nutrition. Most ice cream is delicious and poisonous. Since 1960, water pollution laws have pushed cheese companies to find new disposal systems for whey. Our stomachs are the ideal solution, providing a cheap way to increase milk solids at the minimum level allowed by law. Dr. Philip G. Keeney, Department of Dairy Science, Penn State University, commented, "Nobody uses whey for positive reasons. They use it because it's cheap and it's allowed." Whey has a metallic flavor that a buzzard wouldn't like, but enough sugar and artificial flavor will cover anything. Dr. Keeney concluded, "In a way, ice cream has become the sewage treatment plant of the cheese industry." See this excerpt from *The Raw Truth About Milk*:

And here is the bad part: when you order a banana split at your neighborhood ice cream parlor, you may get vanilla flavored ice cream, chocolate, and strawberry. But you will probably get iporonal (a lice killer) for vanilla, amylphenyl acetate for chocolate, and a solvent called benzyl acetate for strawberry. The toppings will probably be aldehyde C-17 for cherry, ethyl acetate for pineapple (ethyl acetate vapors cause lung, liver, and heart damage), rutyraldehyde for nut flavor, and a paint solvent called amyl acetate for that great banana flavor. It's all economics. Aldehyde C-17 cost seven cents per gallon of ice cream. Real cherries cost thirty-five cents a gallon.

...There are over a thousand different chemicals used in commercial ice cream. How about those beautiful colors added to ice cream to make your birthday memorable? You will get tartrazine (yellow) to upset your stomach, dissamine red 6B for red, and indiotine for blue. You can also be poisoned with ponceau2R, and titanium dioxide.

...Who knows? Maybe you had a titanium deficiency anyway... Coal tar dyes are the major source of artificial coloring. Many of them are known to be potent cancer-causing agents...A single ice cream may contain as many as fifty-five chemical ingredients. If you go really cheap, you might get refiner's syrup as the "nutritive sweetener." Refiner's syrup is the last liquid product of the sugar refining process. It has been described by technicians in the field as "practically inedible."

...You need a good emulsifier to make ice cream. It gives it a characteristic stiffness and richness. They use diethylglycol, and anti-freeze, and polyoxyethylene, which is suspected of causing cancer. They also use polysorbate 65. It deceives you into thinking that the ice cream has a high cream content. As a thickener you may find dioctyl sodium sulfosuccinate, which is a chemical used in medicine as a stool softener (just in case you needed it). One of the most common additives to ice cream is carageenin. When this chemical is added to water and fed to guinea pigs, they develop ulcers. Some scientists think it may cause ulcerative colitis in humans."

...Commercial ice cream is loaded with sugar. Sugar causes diabetes, and according to Dr. Norman Kretchner of Stanford University, sugar is a major cause of atherosclerosis. A person with hypoglycemia (low blood pressure) may faint or have a convulsion from eating sugar-laden commercial ice cream. The convulsions may be from the sugar, or the chemicals, or both.

We could tell you about the additive CMC causing tumors and polysorbate-80 causing premature death in experimental animals, but I guess you get the message:

If you want to go on an Eskimo pie in the sky trip, eat commercial ice cream.

Something else you should know. Unlike milk, there are no federal standards setting the maximum number of bacteria to be allowed in ice cream. They really get away with murder when they sell you "reworked" ice cream. "Reworked" is a euphemism for covering up stale ice cream and selling it as fresh. They just throw it back with the fresh, add more chemicals, and presto—America's fun food. The best way to disguise the poor quality of reworked ice cream is to add a lot of chocolate.

There's not much good news about chocolate. I will touch this subject in a later chapter.

However, if you still want to enjoy ice cream, you can make it yourself, and it is very simple to do. Take two overly ripe bananas (with brown spots), peel them, cut in small slices, and put them in the freezer. A few hours later, take them out, put them in your blender (I use Vita-mix), add a tiny bit of water, and blend. I use the tamper (it's the stick you put through the lid of the blender) and push the bananas around till they get into one creamy mass. You can add vanilla, or frozen blueberries for a different flavor. No sugar needed; the ice-cream will be super sweet and creamy. I usually put bananas in the freezer the day before I intend on making ice cream. For toppings, you can take overly ripe strawberries, wash them, and throw in the blender (frozen strawberries work too). I also use the tamper to push the berries around till they are in a thick liquid mass. I pour it on top of my ice cream, and it's ready to be enjoyed. It's very simple to make it, and it's the healthiest version of ice cream that you can find.

Some deadly reasons why

not to eat meat

The following is an excerpt from the extensively researched book, *The Undigestible Truth About Meat* by Dr. Gina Shaw, M.A., A.I.Y.S.:

"Did you know that the two leading causes of death in the U.S. are directly related to the consumption of meat? When I use the term 'meat,' in order to clear up any confusion anyone may have, I am referring to all animal flesh, be it from cows, turkeys, pigs, chickens, fish, in fact, any animal that lives and breathes and that humans consume! I am talking about all animal flesh."

David Klein, Ph.D., explores this further. See this excerpt from his blog, titled "36 Ways We Damage Our Small Intestine" (and try telling yourself that eating meat is still a good idea!):

Patrice Green, J.D., M.D. and Allison Lee Solin state that animal products easily account for our largest intake of pesticides and herbicides, in fact, more than 80 to 90% by some estimates. Meat also has antibiotic residues. One half of all antibiotics in the US alone are used in the production of livestock. Antibiotics, too, can contribute to hormone-disruptor exposure.

As if that's not enough, in a recent article entitled "Meat Your Death?" by Lawrence J. Jacobs, M.D. and Caroline Kweller, they report that a survey by Public Citizen, the Government Accountability Project, and the American Federation of Government Employees, found that only 46% of federal inspectors had been unable to recall meat laden with animal feces, vomit, metal shards, and other contamination.

In 1998 USDA (United States Department of Agriculture) declared safe for human consumption animal carcasses carrying a host of diseases, such as cancers, tumors, open sores, poultry pneumonia, infection arthritis, and diseases caused by intestinal worms.

Food borne diseases such as campylobacter, listeria, E. coli, and salmonella affect millions of Americans and Britons each year and kill more than 5,000, particularly children, the elderly, and those with weak immune systems. In the vast majority of cases, people contract these diseases after eating animal products such as meat, poultry, eggs, and dairy of from items contaminated by animal products of animal feces.

Animal food is highly acid-forming and, according to Dr. Robert Young, a microbiologist and nutritionist from the

U.S., has high levels of bacteria, yeast/fungus and associated toxins.

Cooked animal foods are dead, enzymatically speaking. They lack enzymes that help us to break down foodstuff, they lack phytonutrients which are by their very nature abundant in fresh, raw plant foods, and they lack many essential vitamins and minerals.

In a recent report by Dr. Green and Ms. Solin, they argue that organic meat, dairy and eggs certainly can't be held to be a healthy option as not only do animal products contain cholesterol, and are typically high in fat, they have been found to significantly raise risks for heart disease, stroke, hypertension, obesity, and cancer.

Meat is the most putrefactive of all foods. This means that meat is more liable to decay in the human gastrointestinal tract than any other food. Flesh, when it is eaten by humans, tends to undergo a process of decay in the stomach or intestinal tract causing a poisoning of the blood. Putrefaction in meat-eaters is evident by bad breath, heartburn, eructations and smelly stools, and it is probable that the attempts of the body to eliminate these wastes has a profound influence on the shortening of our life span.

If the body fluid that bathes our cells is overloaded with waste, an excessive secretion of bile, fatigue, weakening and aging are the inevitable results. The accumulation of toxic substances in the body causes the deterioration of the intestinal flora and the blood vessels gradually lose their natural elasticity, their walls become hardened and thickened. Irreversible damage to the organism will then inevitably occur.

The hardest thing for the human body to digest is cooked animal protein—it leaves us feeling very weak and tired. Protein, being the most complex of all food elements, makes its utilization the most complicated. Those people with impaired digestion will find it preferable to ingest a lesser quantity of concentrated protein which they will be more capable of utilizing, rather than a greater quantity which not only cannot be processed efficiently, but which may poison the body.

When protein is eaten in greater amounts than the body is capable of utilizing, the organism is subjected to the toxic byproducts of protein metabolism, which it has been unable to eliminate—and the inevitable result is degenerative disease. Meat passes very slowly through the human digestive system, which is not designed to digest it in the first place. In fact, flesh foods can take about five days to pass out of the body (plant foods take about one day, at most). During this time the disease-causing products of decaying meat are in constant contact with the digestive organs. The habit of eating animal flesh in its characteristic state of decomposition creates a poisonous state in the colon and wears out the intestinal tract prematurely.

Often, poisonous bacteria present in flesh foods are not destroyed by cooking, especially if the meat is undercooked, barbecued, or roasted on a spit—these are notorious sources of infection. The stomach will attempt to break down animal flesh with chemicals, which are ill-equipped to handle flesh foods as we have a low amount of hydrochloric acid, as compared to carnivorous animals. This hydrochloric acid that we do have is also low in acidity, as compared to a carnivorous animal (20 times less acidic than carnivores).

Next, the animal flesh passes into the small intestine until it comes to the ileocecal valve. Passing through the ileoceacal valve, it enters the cecum, which is at the base of the ascending colon. From here on, the second stage of digestion starts. The chyme becomes a seething mass of intestinal flora. When dead bodies are incorporated in our food, the flora is putrefactive and their mission is to destroy. From the colon, they are drawn into the bloodstream by suction and, as they circulate around the body, disease or sickness is the inevitable result. On a fruit and vegetation diet, the natural flora are fermentative and break down this type of food—they are not pathogenic and are quite harmless to the body for the simple reason that we are not flesh eaters.

British and American scientists who have studied intestinal bacteria of meat-eaters as compared to vegetarians have found significant differences. The bacteria of meat-eaters have been found to cause bowel cancer. This may explain why cancer of the bowel is very prevalent in meat-eating areas like North America and Western Europe, while it is extremely rare in vegetarian countries such as in India. In the US, bowel cancer is the second most common form of cancer (second only to lung cancer). Conversely, recent studies have found that chicken meat is the most carcinogenic meat that people can eat due to the amount of the carcinogen PhIP contained in it— although, as we will find, all meat is dangerous and carcinogenic to the human body.

RawFoodExplained makes another important point: meat contains waste products that were not yet expelled by the animal before it was slaughtered. When the animal dies, all of those toxic fluids, matter, and hormones are released into the cells and tissues. As the body starts to deterioate, cells will continue to release waste materials, trapping them within the bloodstream and an array of damaged tissues. These nitrogenous extracts become trapped, and they contribute to the overall flavor of the meat once cooked.

Waste products are not the only concern. Both before and during the sheer agony of slaughter, the animal is terrified and undergoes profound biochemical changes (just like humans do). Hormone levels skyrocket as the animal fights for its life, and as it sees other animals around it being killed. High hormone levels stay within the muscles and are transferred into your body when you consume their meat.

Dr. David Klein goes in-depth into the devastating side effects of this process in his book, *Self Health Colitis & Crohns*. See the excerpt below for a longer discussion on what happens when we consume meat:

According to the Nutrition Institute of America, "the flesh of an animal carcass is loaded with toxic blood and other waste byproducts." Therefore, toxic byproducts are forced throughout the body, thus poisoning the entire carcass. The flesh is invaded by putrefactive viruses, which are nature's scavengers that function to get rid of dead bodies. As soon as an animal is killed, proteins in its body coagulate, and self-destructive enzymes are released (unlike slow decaying plants which have a rigid cell wall). Soon denatured substances called ptomaines are formed. Due to these ptomaines that are released immediately after death, animal flesh and eggs have a common property: extremely rapid decomposition and putrefaction. By the time the animal is slaughtered, placed in cold storage, "aged," transported to the butcher's shop or supermarket and purchased, brought home, stored, prepared, and eaten, one can imagine what stage of decay one's dinner is in. According to the Encyclopedia Britannica, body poisons, including uric acid and other toxic wastes, are present in the blood and tissue.

Cholesterol is mainly found in animal products. Meat, fish, poultry, dairy products and eggs, etc., all contain cholesterol, while plant products, on the whole, do not. Choosing lean cuts of meat is not enough, the cholesterol is mainly in the lean portion. Many people are surprised to learn that chicken contains as much cholesterol as beef. Every four-ounce serving of beef or chicken contains 100 milligrams of cholesterol. Most shellfish are very high in cholesterol. There is no "good cholesterol" in any food.

Colon cancer is acknowledged to be among one of the predominant type of cancer in the United States. It is the second leading cause of cancer mortality. An article in the *Wall Street Journal* several years ago tells about a study of colon cancer by Dr. William Haenzel, Dr. John W. Berg and others at the National Cancer Institute. Dr. Berg said: "There is now substantial evidence that beef is a key factor in determining bowel cancer incidence."

Scientists have reported evidence that two characteristics of meat-based diets are specific influences in colon cancer: 1) Fecal transit time—a low-fiber diet allows carcinogens to be concentrated and held in contact with the bowel mucosa for long periods, while a high residue diet (a vegetarian diet) produces more rapid passage of body waste, 2) Influence of the diet on the amount of carcinogens produced by the body: it has been found that meat has tends toward production of carcinogens in the intestine.

Let us now examine the charge that flesh-eating is supposed to be a superior source of protein. Well, upon examining the evidence, the truth is exactly opposite!

The effects of encumbering our bodies with the proteins of other animals serve to promote diseased conditions of the human organism. Dr. Herbert M. Shelton wrote that allergy and anaphylaxis (a kind of toxic shock of the tissues) are not mysterious and that they are due to long-standing poisoning of the body by excess or inappropriate protein foods. Animal proteins are often not reduced to their constituent amino acids, but are absorbed in more complex form. Absorption by the body of such partially digested proteins poison the human body and so-called "allergic symptoms may result in gout, arthritis, cancer, or any one or more host of degenerative diseases.

One of the favorite arguments of flesh-eaters is that proteins from the plant kingdom are "incomplete," because, they say, no plant food contains all of the twenty-three identical amino acids. Studies of man's physiology and the effect of his consumption of foods from plant kingdom have shown conclusively that it is not necessary to consume all of the amino acids in one sitting, or even the eight (some references say ten) essential amino acids that are not fabricated within the body. Foods we eat are processed by the body, and the amino acids, vitamins, minerals, and other nutrients are reserved in a pool for later use as needed. When we eat, we replenish the reserves in this pool, which is then drawn upon by cells as and when required. We do not live upon one protein food, but upon the protein content of our varied diet, which provides all of the protein needs of the body. Guyton's *Guidance Textbook of Medical Physiology* is authority to this important information. The book shows that amino acids are picked up from the bloodstream and cells of the body.

Dr. Hoobler, researching at Yale University, demonstrated the superiority of nut protein. It was he who proved conclusively that the protein of nuts not only provides greater nutritive efficiency than that of meat, milk and eggs, but that it is also more effective than a combination of these three animal proteins. Fruits and vegetables, although containing relatively smaller amounts of protein in their natural state, are excellent sources of amino acids for complete and optimal nutrition as well. The protein in raw nuts and seeds [sprouted/soaked] and in uncooked fruits and vegetables, are readily available to the body, and are therefore said to be of high biological value. During the process of digestion, the long chains of amino acids (the building blocks of protein) are gradually broken up for the body's use in synthesizing its own protein (as any species must do).

However, when proteins have been cooked or preserved, they are coagulated. Enzyme resistant linkages are formed that resist cleavage, and the amino acids may not be released for body use. In this case, the protein is useless and/or poisonous to the body, becoming soil for bacteria and a poisonous decomposition byproduct.

Since the nutrients available from raw food are several hundred % greater than those available from food that has been cooked or otherwise processed, and since flesh foods are usually not eaten raw and whole by humans, this in itself would be an important reason why firsthand protein foods from the plant kingdom, which may be eaten uncooked, are superior.

...Nowadays, many people eat fish rather than beef in the hope of limiting fat and cholesterol; however, many fish including catfish, swordfish, and sea trout contain almost one-third fat (saturated fat also contributes to degenerative disease). In fact, salmon is 52% fat and, ounce for ounce, shrimps have double the cholesterol of beef. The Physicians Committee for Responsible Medicine argue that fish and fish oil capsules contain an unhealthy amount of artery-clogging saturated fat and that, studies show that diets based on fish do nothing to reverse arterial blockages. Moreover, blockages continue to worsen for patients who regularly eat fish. Fortunately, eating vegetables such as broccoli, lettuce and beans provides essential fatty acids in a more stable form, with zero cholesterol and little saturated fat, which are a much healthier substitute!

Contrary to the myths that chicken and turkey (and fish) contain less cholesterol and that, reportedly, chicken and turkey represent a good option for those on a healthier diet, Dean Ornish, M.D., reported that on a five-year follow-up of patients on his popular plan for reversing heart disease with a totally vegetarian diet, compared with patients on the chicken and fish diet recommended by the American Heart Association (AHA), the majority following the AHA guidelines got progressively worse, whilst those who made intensive changes got progressively better.

Kieswer stated that too much protein also puts a strain on the kidneys, forcing them to expel extra nitrogen in the urine, increasing the risk for kidney disease. Also, the combination of fat, protein and carcinogens found in cooked chicken creates troubling risks for colon cancer.

Chicken not only gives you a load of fat you don't want, its heterocyclic amines (HCAs) are potent carcinogens produced from creatine, amino acids and sugars in poultry and other meats during cooking. These same chemicals are found in tobacco smoke and are 15 times more concentrated in grilled chicken than in beef. HCAs may be one of the reasons that meat-eaters have much higher colon cancer rates, about 300% higher compared to vegetarians.

Dr. Neal Barnard of the Physicians Committee for Resposible Medicine, in reviewing recent research findings, stated that it has long been known that cooked red meat contains cancer-causing heterocyclic amines, which form as the meat is heated, but the U.S. National Cancer Institue has shown that oven-broiled, pan-fried or grilled/barbecued chicken carries an even bigger load of these carcinogens than does red meat. In fact, they argue that chicken is far more cancer-causing than red meat (the number of PhIPs in a well-done steak contains about 30 ng/g, but grilled chicken reached 480 ng/g). These dangerous chemicals are strongly linked to colon cancer, but may also contribute to breast cancer. Conversely, Dr. Barnard also mentions that the cholesterol content of chicken is actually the same as that of beef, and the fat content is not much different either.

So, to recap all the mentioned info above, let's go over all the deadly reasons why it's best to stay away from eating animal flesh.

1) All meat is FULL OF CHEMICALS. You may have heard this argument before: that eating meat is simply being "on the top of the food chain." But there's more to the chain than animals eating other animals. After all, plants "eat" the sunlight, the air, and the water. Fields that are treated with poisonous chemicals, such as pesticides and fertilizers, are used as feeding grounds for animals that consume grasses and plants. One example is DDT, a powerful insect-killing chemical that also happens to be linked to cancer, serioius liver diseases, and even

sterility in humans. If an animal eats grasses or
grains that have been treated with DDT, that
pesticide will stay in their bodies (even in fish).
That means any pesticide or fertilizer is passed
along to you—and just think about all of the
harmful chemicals and poison that the animal
has ingested throughout its lifetime. (And
believe me, those animals were not fed "top
organic" grass, they are fed toxic waste just to
fatten them up so they are ready to be killed for
you.)

If you're eating at the "top" of the food
chain, that means that you become the final
resting link on that chain and are consuming
the highest concentration of chemicals,
pesticides, and poison. In fact, No2Meat claims
that "meat contains 13 times more DDT than
vegetables, fruits and grass."

Scientific research supports this claim.
According to Civil Eats: "Researchers at the
Johns Hopkins Center for a Livable Future
published a study in the scientific journal
Environmental Health Perspectives that
provided further evidence of the risks

associated with the use of arsenicals in animal agriculture. The study, which involved analysis of chicken breast samples purchased at grocery stores in 10 cities across the US, revealed that chickens, likely raised with arsenic-based drugs, yield meat that has higher levels of inorganic arsenic, a known carcinogen that has also been associated with cardiovascular diseases, type 2 diabetes, cognitive deficits and adverse pregnancy outcomes."

2) Meats are FULL OF DISEASES. There is even more poison to consider in meat. Animals are given hormones and chemicals to make them grow faster and bigger, put fat on their bones, and even to boost the color of their meat. Animals are force-fed, given stimulants to boost their appetite, and are even given sedatives, antibiotics, and chemicals in the foods that they consume. These chemicals have been scientifically proven to be linked to cancer, and there are plenty of animals that die before they even enter the slaughter room. Farms are now simply meat factories, and animal welfare is the least of their concern.

Many animals are never given the opportunity to exercise, graze, or even get a few minutes of fresh air. Instead, they spend their lives in cages and in cramped areas. This mistreatment alters their natural body chemistry, changing their day-to-day routines and creating deformities such as tumors.

These tumors are incredibly common in the US. As many as 90% of cattle are on an antibiotic regimen—and even with medical treatment, there are millions of pounds of tumors that are hidden within the meat that is packaged and sold. In some cases, these growths might slip by unnoticed—but there are other cases where inspectors and farmers have outright ignored their presence in order to turn a profit. Even if a tumor is spotted, all it takes to produce a "high-quality" cut of meat is to remove the tumor and carry on, letting the rest of the cancerous cells remain. (This is incredibly easy to do in hot dogs). Experiments have shown that if a fish eats the liver of an animal that had cancer, the fish will also get cancer.

3) Meats are FULL OF BODY TOXINS. Don't forget about all of the biochemical changes that occur before, during, and after an animal is slaughtered. All of those hormones and waste products are sent throughout the animal's cells, bloodstream, and muscles, spreading poison. The Nutrition Institute of America supports this, saying that an animal carcass contains flesh that is filled with waste.

This has significant consequences for human health over the long term. According to EliasOriano.com: "About 5% of the flesh volume of all animals consists of waste material called uric acid that is normally eliminated by the kidneys. Uric acid is poisonous to humans, because it is toxic and non-metabolizable. Nearly 100% of Americans suffer some form of osteoporosis that is due in large part, to the acidic end-products of meat (and dairy, grain, and processed foods) eating. All carnivorous animals however, secrete the enzyme uricase that breaks down uric acid so it can be readily eliminated."

Humans generate only enough uricase to deal with uric acid that is produced during a normal day of metabolizing. As a result, the human body will absorb uric acid when meat is eaten; then, calcium-urate crystals form and concentrate in joints, feet, and in the lower back. These deposits lead to arthritis, gout, rheumatism, bursitis, and lower back pain. As Elias Oriano so succinctly says, "Humans are physiologically unsuited to utilizing meat as food."

I would suggest you conduct an experiment. Take a piece of meat, chew it, and then spit it out on the plate, and leave it on the table at a room temperature. The next morning, you will find a rotting peace of flesh that won't be appealing at all. That is exactly what is happening inside of you. You just can't see it, but it's the same end result — putrefaction inside of you, and it takes two to three days (even up to five days) till that toxic flesh exits your system.

4) Meats are FULL OF DECAY. Any meat that is raw will be constantly decaying.

Once the animal is slaughtered, ptomaines start to form. These denatured substances are immediately released once the animal dies, and they promote rapid decomposition of the flesh. It takes a very long time for meat to go through our digestive system (yet another sign that we are not meant to be meat-eaters). In total, it can take anywhere between two to five days for meat to go through your digestive system. In that time, the decaying meat is in hours upon hours of contact with your organs, wearing down the colon and the intestinal tract.

5) Meats are FULL OF BACTERIA. The E coli 0157 bacteria, a strain of life-threatening bacteria that can cause body diarrhea and dehydration, is naturally present in the intestines of cattle. Time and again, ground beef products in the US have been found to be contaminated with bacteria. There was a case in the past when some 1.1 million pounds of ground beef caused 22 cases of illness in Minnesota. According to the U.S. National Centers for disease control in 2001 report, the products were believed to have been

contaminated with both E coli 0157 and salmonella combined to sicken at least 113,000 people annually. Those who are very young and those who are very old (and anyone who is immuno-compromised) are significantly more at risk to E coli and any related illnesses.

Even if you eat your meat well-done, you are still at risk. Meat that is cooked at a high temperature can stimulate the production of chemicals that have been linked to breast cancer, stomach cancer, and colon cancer. Heterocyclicamines (HCAs) are produced when meat is cooked at high temperatures, such as broiling, frying, and grilling. Polycyclic aromatic hydrocarbons (PAHs) are transferred through flame and smoke, making your dinner just as harmful as smoking a whole pack of cigarettes at once.

6) Meats are FULL OF FATS AND CHOLESTEROL. Beef, poultry, lamb, and pork have tons of saturated fat (and factory-farmed animals have even more). The amount of meat that a population eats has a direct affect on overall lifespan. Take, for example, research

from John Robbins in his book, *Diet for a New America*:

"The cultures with the very longest life spans in the world are the Vilcambas, who reside in the Andes of Ecuador, the Abkhasians, who live on the Black Sea in the USSR, and the Hunzas, who live in the Himalayas of Northern Pakistan. Researchers discovered a "striking similarity" in the diets of these groups, scattered though they are in different parts of the planet. All three are either totally vegetarian or close to it. The Hunzas, who are the largest of the three groups, eat almost no animal products. Meat and dairy products combined account for only 1.5% of their total calories."

7) Meats are FULL OF GENETICALLY ALTERED SUBSTANCES. While we haven't yet started raising herds of genetically modified animals, there is plenty of opportunity for animals to be poisoned by GMOs. Soy, potatoes, and corn are all genetically modified and given to cows and other farm animals. These genetically modified foods can result in

respiratory issues, nausea, rashes, and even death. When animals eat genetically modified foods and then pass those chemicals along to humans, the pesticide and chemicals are transferred in a much more concentrated form.

The reason they are so highly concentrated is because they build up as one organism passes the chemicals along to another. Pesticides and other poisonous contaminants are stored within body fat; this can occur even if an animal is only exposed to pesticides and doesn't ingest them.

For anyone who wants to know another 100 reasons supported by the researches and proof why animal products are bad for you (if you are still not convinced), I suggest reading *The China Study: The Most Comprehensive Study of Nutrition Ever Conducted And the Startling Implications for Diet, Weight Loss, And Long-term Health* written by T. Colin Campbell, Ph.D. Dr. T. Colin Campbell has more than four decades of nutrition research and experience. *The China Study* has been widely regarded as the most comprehensive study of health and nutrition ever conducted.

Dr. Campbell gave us a simple but powerful answer: "Eat a diet based on whole, plant-based food, and dramatically reduce your risk of a broad spectrum of diseases, including heart disease, obesity, diabetes, and cancer." He provides statistics and data on correlation of animal products vs human health conditions, and based on all that information you can come to your own conclusion that any animal products are very harmful to our health.

What do I eat instead of meat? Before I transitioned to fruitarian lifestyle, I was vegan for a brief time, and then also a raw vegan. Despite what you might be thinking, there *is* plant protein that is more suitable for us than meat protein. You can find it in fruits and veggies. It was easier on my body than on my mind. Societal conditioning that life is impossible without meat was haunting me for a while, especially with my father's lectures (after all, he is a doctor) on "How it's impossible to survive and be healthy without meat." I realized that there are a few options that were suitable for me and I loved them: broccoli, avocado (which is a fruit), and chlorella (but be careful with this one—it is a strong detoxifier for heavy metals, so you should start very slow on this one). There are also awesome seeds that I used occasionally for protein such as chia seeds, flax seeds, and hemp seeds—they are all great sources of Omegas 3,6,9, and a great substitute for fish as well.

Personally, I ate a lot of broccoli every day when I was transitioning into raw foods. I ate a plate of broccoli a day (not cooked all the way, but close to raw). I was loading up on it till I realized that it became too heavy for me, and then I started looking for something lighter. But it was a big portion of my diet during the transition.

Avocados provide all 18 essential amino acids necessary for the body to form a complete protein, plus seven fatty acids, including Omega 3 and 6. Unlike the protein in steak, which is difficult for most people to digest, avocado protein is readily absorbed by the body, because avocadoes also contain fiber. If you are trying to cut down on animal sources of protein in your diet, or if you are a vegetarian or vegan seeking more protein, avocados are a great nutritional ally to include not merely as an occasional treat, but as a regular part of your diet.

I was personally loading up on avocados every day when I switched to a fruitarian lifestyle. Later in my progression (when my body became cleaner), I realized that avocados were starting to become too heavy for me. At first I cut down to half of an avocado a day (when I started the transition, initially, I would load up on three to four avocados daily), and then I stopped eating them all together (along with seeds and nuts, which also became too heavy for me).

The thing is, when you are toxic, your absorption is 5% of all the foods that you consume, so you have to eat 10 times more in order not to stay hungry. To simplify the idea, your receptors are blocked with toxins like a cork in a bottle, and the toxins won't let any nutrients to be absorbed. The toxins are like a cork, a solid barrier.

Moreover, some toxins mimic nutrients and minerals and while your body is malnourished, it is fooled by toxins that you have enough of this or that mineral or vitamin. For example, lead mimics calcium, and attaches to the receptors where calcium is supposed to be. Your body kind of functions, but in reality you are calcium deficient; however, all the spaces where calcium is supposed to go is taken by lead (which is a heavy metal toxin), and it won't allow calcium to replace it. No matter how many calcium supplements you take, it will just go through you and exit the body without any effect. To increase your absorption, you have to detox lead. Once lead is removed from your system, the calcium can be freely replenished. As you detox and get cleaner, your absorption increases, so you don't need to eat much at all. Your food consumption decreases dramatically.

The last main source of protein for me was chlorella. I was making sure I was getting organically grown, broken wall cell chlorella. They are pressed into small green pills. I started with one pill a day, and eventually worked up to 20 a day. That's pretty much all the protein you need for the day if you weigh about 100 lbs.

There are also a lot of other options for your source of protein; all greens are a great source of protein, among other fruits like jackfruit, which I love, but it's seasonal. Durian is another great source of protein: it's a dense fruit, so you can really get full eating it. I can't name all the options, but I know they are endless if you look into it and do a little research. With such a wide array of options in the plant kingdom, you can definitely find the best veggies and fruits for your tastes and preferences.

Is fish bad for you?

Fish that have been raised on a farm and fed high-grain diets have high amounts of omega 6, a fatty acide that actually promotes inflammation. In fact, catfish and tilapia that eat corn and soy pellets are much more unhealthy than you think. Their diet can cause them to have more fat than bacon, hamburgers, or doughnuts. And those pellets are probably GMO, as there is no NON-GMO corn left in the US. About 90% of corn is GMO that has non-organic pesticides.

People don't realize that GMO and organic are two different stories, and they are surprised that GMO veggie or fruit can be grown without the use of pesticides, which will automatically make it organic. From my personal experience of talking to a person that works at one of the grocery health stores, I learned that organic and non-organic fruits and veggies often get mixed up (by US law, it's illegal to have organic produce GMO, but for some reason I highly doubt that this law is closely followed or inspected).

Besides, larger fish like marlin contain so much mercury that they're dangerous for pregnant women and children to eat due to the potential for developmental disorders. Even regular people can develop memory problems, tremors, vision trouble, and more. Now that eating fish is encouraged as a healthy protein source laden with desirable omega-3 fatty acids, people must be more concerned than ever with contamination from hydrocarbons, noxious chemicals, radiation, and heavy metals poisoning from mercury, cadmium and arsenic.

Radiation is a huge issue, especially after the Fukashima nuclear disaster. I strongly recommend you Google this issue; I bet you will never touch fish again if you live in Northern America. Scientists say that although hydrocarbons in the Gulf of Mexico are carcinogenic, they do eventually break down over time, allowing for the dissolution of contaminants. This does not mean those fish are safe to eat, but at least there is hope.

However, mercury and other heavy metals in fish may still remain in the food chain indefinitely, with no one knowing how long it will take for those fish to be really safe to eat.

Mercury is a toxic heavy metal and is considered one of the most dangerous poisons on earth. It has been found to contaminate many inland waterways in the US to some degree, according to reports from *Scientific American* and The U.S. Geological Survey. Findings of a study were reported in August 2009 after 291 rivers and streams were tested between 1998 to 2005. The study found that 75% of all fish in these streams had detectable amounts of mercury, and 25% had dangerous levels, above what is considered safe for human consumption. According to a recent study by Got Mercury?, a San Francisco-based public awareness campaign, mercury levels in California's store-bought fish are sky-high.

The Turtle Island Restoration Network, which runs the campaign, said it tested 98 samples of fish from randomly selected grocery stores throughout California. It found that all

98 samples contained detectable amounts of mercury. The biggest culprits are: 81% of swordfish samples that registered high levels of mercury (nine of those samples were more than 200 times over the maximum acceptable levels set by federal food safety officials); and 20% of the tuna sushi samples were over the mercury action level determined by the U.S. Food and Drug Administration (USFDA).

Fewer than half of the stores posted signs advising pregnant women not to eat swordfish and other fish high in mercury. Overall, one third of the fish samples were found to contain levels of mercury exceeding the USFDA's mercury action level (1 part per million).

One of the simple solutions for substitution of all Omegas (as well as omitting eating fish) is flax seeds. Flax seed plays three primary roles in nutrition: 1) Flax seed is high in soluble and insoluble dietary fiber, making it a great dietary aid; 2) Flax seed is a great source of lignans, which is a nutrient that acts as an antioxidant to fight free radicals in the body; 3) Flax seed is highly concentrated with Omega-3 fatty acids. Omega-3 is the fatty acid that is most often missing from the Standard American Diet.

You can make raw dehydrated bread/crackers with flax seeds. Add one cup of flax seeds, then add three peeled, sliced apples (apples go first). Put everything in the blender. Add a dash of cinnamon and salt, blend, and put in a dehydrator at 98°F overnight and the bread is ready. You can find all sorts of flax seed bread recipes on Youtube, including flax seed bread for sandwiches and flax seed bread for tea. Also, you can eat flax seeds by themselves or put them on green salad. You can add a tablespoon of flax seeds to smoothies (preferably savory smoothies, not sweet ones). Also, I learned that flax seed oil helps with the symptoms of allergies and are a great digestive aid. If you want to regulate your bowels, take one to two tablespoons of flax seed oil daily, and you will never have a problem with constipation.

Instead of eating fish, you can use Chia seeds. Chia seeds can help reduce blood pressure. The seeds contain one of the highest known plant sources of essential fatty acids (Omega-3 and Omega-6). EFAs cannot be synthesized by our bodies (that is what our society believes, at least); however, it is very important that we get enough to support our immune, cardiovascular, nervous, and reproductive systems. EFA deficiency is quite common in North America.

According to Charlotte Bradley on the What's Cooking America website:

Chia seeds slow down the rate at which complex carbohydrates are digested and are then assimilated into the body. The soluble fiber helps to stabilize blood glucose levels resulting in steady, sustained energy. In one study on diabetic patients, Dr. Vladamir Vuksan of St. Michael's Hospital in Toronto, found that blood was thinner, less prone to clotting, and blood pressure of participants dropped significantly, after three months of taking chia seeds daily.

The word "Chia" comes from the Mayan language and means strength. Chia seeds are a balanced blend of protein, carbohydrates, fats, and fiber. It is said that 1 tablespoon of Chia can sustain a person for 24 hours. Athletes have reported that Chia seeds help them perform at optimal levels for much longer periods of time.

A number of arthritis sufferers notice reduced pain and inflammation after a few weeks of taking Chia seeds. The high concentration of omega-3 helps to lubricate joints and keep them supple. Additionally, Omega-3s are converted into prostaglandins, which are known to have both pain relieving, and anti-inflammatory effects.

The essential fatty acids contained in Chia seeds helps to boost metabolism and promote lean muscle mass. The seeds are sometimes added to food to provide bulk and nutrients while adding very few calories. For these reasons, many people have found Chia quite useful in weight loss and weight maintenance.

Similar to psyllium, the swelling action of Chia in the body helps to cleanse and soothe the colon and absorb toxins while lubricating and strengthening peristaltic action.

Chia seeds contain about 20% protein, a higher percentage than normally found in many other grains such as wheat and rice. Chia seeds contain strontium, which helps to assimilate protein and produce high energy.

Chia seeds are also an excellent source of antioxidants containing even more antioxidants than fresh blueberries. The high amounts of antioxidants in Chia seeds also keeps the oils from going rancid thus, contributing to a long shelf life.

Besides EFAs, Chia seeds also provide fiber, iron, calcium, niacin, magnesium, zinc, and phosphorus. Two tablespoons of Chia is equal to 7 grams of fiber, 2 grams of protein, 205 milligrams of calcium, and 5 grams of omega-3.

EFAs are known to make cell membranes more flexible and efficient, making nutrients more readily available and nerve transmission more efficient. This helps to improve brain function (including memory and concentration).

In addition to that, if you have an upset stomach and gas, the best way to fix it is to eat a tablespoon of dry chia seeds with a small glass of water. Once they are in your stomach, they will absorb all the toxic materials and brewing liquids in your system, which will give you relief within 20 minutes.

Eggs

You would think that eggs are good for you—after all, they have tons of protein and vitamin D, and they're so often added to salads and our breakfast meals. The truth is that eggs are poison in your body. As stated in an article titled "7 Foods You Eat That Are Actually Poison" on *Thought Catalog*: "A recent study found that eggs are about as bad for you as smoking in terms of heart disease, increasing carotid wall thickness (a standard measure for heart disease risk) by nearly as much as someone who smokes regularly."

It makes sense since even a single egg yolk has 200mg of cholesterol and the daily intake limit is 300mg. In addition, no one I know eats only one egg at breakfast. As the Mayo Clinic reportedly says, "Chicken eggs are high in cholesterol, and a diet high in cholesterol can contribute to high blood cholesterol levels."

Eggs are constipating and mucus-forming. They will clog your intestines. Also, if you were not introduced with the idea of eating a bird's embryo, would this idea sound weird to you if you had just learned about it? Some people think it's weird to eat sea-urchin, or fish "eggs" called caviar, but some people eat them from childhood and find them completely normal.

Other cultures like to eat bull testicles, but if you were offered to eat them, would it sound strange to you? So, why eating raw eggs doesn't turn you off? You will reply that you want them to be cooked for you. But through cooking we destroy everything that was useful in the egg to our bodies. We are left with literally "plastic" and cholesterol, with a dash of toxins to eat.

I missed eggs when I gave them up, and I was craving them for a while. It was easier for me to give up meat, but eggs were difficult. I was craving the taste, but soon enough the cravings stopped. Within a year, I felt like I was craving eggs again and decided to give in (after all, I hadn't had eggs in more than a year). So, I went out and ordered eggs. I was looking forward to eating them. But, to my surprise, when I tried them, after abstaining from them for so long, they tasted like some rotten, weird thing. I couldn't eat them.

I was very surprised and puzzled. Once your body purifies itself, your senses become much more heightened and refined. Your taste buds become more sensitive. What you haven't noticed before, you sure will notice now. So, after that experiment of egg-tasting, I never reverted back to eating them again. When I was passing by a breakfast café where they served eggs, they smelled good from a distance, but I knew that it was a deceptive association of old conditioning through the sense of comfort of my experiences that I had before. It is really strange how taste buds change—and along with that, our perceptions and choices in foods change as well.

Protein

I highly recommend you read this priceless book called *Self Healing Colitis & Crohn's* by David Klein, Ph.D. This book is not only for people who experience intestinal problems, but also for anyone who wants to learn why the fruitarian diet is the most optimal for humans. It also explains how our body works, and how it is possible to heal our own bodies with fruits and veggies. If you want to upgrade or improve your health, I would definitely say that this book is worth your time.

In his book, David Klein discusses and explains all that we need to know about protein. See this excerpt for his take on protein:

Protein is one of the two largest dietary concerns (the other being the suitability of fruit), which arise for people considering this vegan diet approach. Concerns and fears are typically rooted in common erroneous beliefs: social conditioning which is based on falsehoods about health and nutrition stemming from at least a century of propaganda propagated by the meat, dairy, and medical industries.

The happy truth about protein is that even the simplest vegan diet is an abundantly sufficient source of superior protein (actually, the building blocks of protein, from which all animals build their protein are amino acids) and we don't have to worry about it except in extreme cases of emaciation. High-protein foods are not needed, not even digestible ones. Fruits and vegetables are premium, sufficient sources of amino acids, the building blocks of protein, which our cells (primarily those of the liver) use to synthesize ALL of its protein. No—the protein in the flesh and muscles of a meat eater and milk drinker is not comprised of the very protein molecules that were ingested. Rather, that protein was synthesized from the amino acids, which were reduced from protein molecules and assimilated after digestion in the small intestine.

Another happy truth is that the body recycles approximately 80% of the protein it makes. As such, we don't need to concern ourselves with eating an abundance of protein every day because we simply don't normally lose much.

Those who believe that they are deriving quality protein from cooked meats are mistaken. The protein from cooked foods is largely destroyed or rendered unusable by the heat. In actuality, very little protein or amino acids are available from meat and dairy or any other cooked foods. Then how is it possible to grow and build muscle if only a little protein is available from meat and dairy?

All our protein needs are provided by plants and their fruits. Synthesis of the eight essential amino acids occurs in plants. Only plants extract nitrogen from the air and nitrates from the soil for amino acid synthesis. Humans and other animals obtain essential amino acids from plant foods, including fruits. Plants and fruits wouldn't exist without amino acids as a part of their structures. The non-essential amino acids are synthesized within our bodies by digestive reduction of more complex amino acids (protein molecules) into simpler amino acids.

A broad diet of plant foods, which excludes any and all animal foods, provides all eight essential amino acids required by the body for all of its protein needs. We will get enough amino acids if we simply eat vegan meals of appropriate foods. Countless vegans have found their new eating style to be more satisfying and beneficial than their previous meat-based diets."

Also, current bone density testing has verified a loss of calcium from the bones after the consumption of just one meat meal. A similar meal containing the same amount of protein from plants results in no calcium loss.

Let's see what facts and fallacies Dr. Douglas Graham discloses about protein:

Although protein was the first nutrient to be discovered and named, most people are still worried about getting enough. This is paradoxical, as shortage of protein is a practically unknown condition. Even through we learned in grammar school Biology, that the nucleus of every living cell contains DNA, which is made out of protein, many people still think that foods such as fruits and vegetables are devoid of protein. This is in-spite of the fact that these same people know full well that there are many species of creatures in nature that live out their life span eating nothing but fruits and veggies.

Dr. T.C. Fry wrote a widely cited article titled "Fruits, Seeds, Nuts, & Fruit Eaters." See the below for an excerpt on human's natural relationship with fruit:

When ripened, fruits accommodatingly covert their carbohydrate components into glucose and fructose, which are simple sugars we can use without further digestion. Their enzymes convert their proteins into amino acids and their fats into fatty acids and glycerols. Fruits supply from 4 to 8 grams of amino acids per 100 grams, almost every one of them with all the essential amino acids in the required proportions for humans, plus, of course, other amino acids.

The average amino acid content is about the same as mother's milk for a growing baby. The average is about 6% of solids.

When sufficient calories have been consumed to meet caloric needs, intake is almost double of that of our actual daily amino acid shortfall from recycling. Furthermore, the fatty acids from almost all fruits other than avocados and olives constitute about 1% to 5% of solids other than fiber. These fatty acids are liberal in their supply of the essential fatty acids. The average fatty acid content of fruits is about 2%. But, more importantly, fruits are rich in mineral matter in the most utilizable form in all of nature! Of its solids, about 3% are minerals including, of course, ample calcium to meet our needs if we don't eat more than 20% acid-forming foods and if we don't cook and derange fruit nutrients.

We don't really need to crunch a great many numbers in order to determine our true protein intake needs. Protein is an essential building block for growth. Human mother's milk averages about 7%

of its calories from protein. This enables an infant to grow at meteoric speed while gaining as much as 12 pounds in just 6 months. It can be safely assumed that adults need no more protein per calorie than an infant, as the adult's growth rate is far slower. Various types of research and countless studies have confirmed that mid-single digit protein consumption, as a function of total calories consumed, is more than enough for our requirements.

Health seekers have fully tested this concept through the use of fasting as a method of healing from injury and disease. While following a "diet" of rest and water, sometimes for 30 or 40 days or even longer, protein deficiency has never been encountered in fasters. The body demonstrated that it had sufficient protein available by successfully working its healing magic during the fasts.

A wide variety of bodily ills are overcome during water fasts, including those that definitely require protein, such as wound and bone healing. This shows that humans carry a large protein reserve of what are called "labile proteins", ones that are not structurally integrated. Therefore, heavy protein consumption is not necessary on a daily basis. In fact, the over consumption of dense protein source foods typically results in harm to one's health.

Fruits and vegetables have long been considered health foods. A diet consisting of nothing but fruits and vegetables will supply a protein content of about 8% per calorie. It has been shown repeatedly that diets supplying double digit protein per calorie consumed, leads to a variety of health problems including heart and vascular disease, kidney disorders, liver dysfunctions, arthritis and a wide variety of cancers. A primary reason for these problems is foods that are rich in protein, are usually also very high in fat. It is rare to find a high protein food that doesn't have fat as its primary source of calories. Certainly this is true of all flesh foods, dairy, nuts, and seeds.

Eating protein doesn't build muscle. Muscular growth results from placing a strength overload upon the muscles and then supplying adequate conditions for recovery. Repeatedly using this overload and recovery strategy results in steady and reliable muscular growth and development. The quality of tissue developed will be determined by the foods eaten. The highest quality tissues will develop as a result of eating fruits and vegetables.

Protein, per se, is not actually used by the body to build new tissue. When foods are eaten, their constituent proteins are broken down during the digestive processes into ever smaller particles; proteoles, polypeptides, dipeptides, and, eventually, amino acids. The amino acids travel to the liver where they are recombined and constructed into the specific proteins needed at any given time.

Not only is it a fallacy that protein will result in muscle growth, but the concept that the body needs specific proteins, from fish, meat, eggs, etc. is also fallacious. The body breaks down all proteins to their component amino acids before recombining them. Eating the muscles from animals will not result in our developing bigger muscles. As an analogy, eating animal's eyes will not improve your vision, nor will eating their brains increase our intellect.

The protein content of fruits and vegetables is prefect for human beings as it is for all of the animals in the

anthropoid family. Gorillas have no
trouble growing big and strong on fruits
and veggies, and the same applies to us.
Don't fall for yet another health-
destroying gimmick. Eat fruits and
veggies with confidence, knowing that
you are supplying yourself with the
world's most nutritious foods.

As you can tell, whole fruits and
vegetables have all of the protein that we
need! And despite what you've been told
your whole life, protein does NOT build
muscle.

Is wheat good for you?

One of the best explanations of what wheat does to your body comes from an article posted on Gizmodo.com, titled "Why you should probably stop eating wheat." See the excerpt below for a deeper discussion on why wheat is depleting your health:

Wheat and grain-based foods are all around us. We love our bagels, pasta, bread, and breakfast cereals. For many, the thought of eliminating these staples from our diets seems wholly unreasonable, if not ludicrous... As science is increasingly showing, eating wheat increases the potential for a surprising number of health problems....

...[Wheat] supplies about 20% of the total food calories worldwide, and is a national staple in most countries. But as is well known, some people, like those with celiac disease, need to stay away from it.

The problem is that their small intestine is unable to properly digest gluten, a protein that is found in grains. But wheat is being increasingly blamed for the onset of other health conditions such as obesity, heart disease, and a host of digestive problems — including the dramatic rise in celiac-like disorders...Wheat raises blood sugar levels, causes immunoreactive problems, inhibits the absorption of important minerals, and aggravates our intestines. And much of this may stem from the fact that wheat simply isn't what it used to be.

Indeed, today's wheat is a far cry from what it used to be 50 years ago. Back in the 1950s, scientists began cross-breeding wheat to make it harder, shorter, and better-growing. This work, which was the basis for the Green Revolution — and one that won U.S. plant scientist Norman Borlaug the Nobel Prize — introduced some compounds to wheat that aren't entirely human friendly.

As cardiologist Dr. William Davis noted in his book, *Wheat Belly: Lose the Wheat, Lose the Weight and Find Your Path Back to Health*, today's hybridized wheat contains sodium azide, a known toxin. It also goes through a gamma irradiation process during manufacturing.

But as Davis also points out, today's hybridized wheat contains novel proteins that aren't typically found in either the parent or the plant, some of which are difficult for us to properly digest. Consequently, some scientists now suspect that the gluten and other compounds found in today's modern wheat is what is responsible for the rising prevalence of celiac disease, "gluten sensitivity", and other problems.

...Gluten is a protein composite of gliadin and glutenin that appears in wheat as well as other grains like rye, barley, and spelt. It's also what gives certain foods that wonderful, chewy texture. Gluten also helps dough to rise and keep its shape. The problem, however, is in how it's metabolized. According to Alessio Fasano, the Medical Director for The University of Maryland's Center for Celiac Research, no one can properly digest gluten. "We do not have the enzymes to break it down," he said in a recent interview with *TenderFoodie*. "It all depends upon how well our intestinal walls close after we ingest it and how our immune system reacts to it." His concern is that the gluten protein, which is abundant in the endosperm of barley, rye, and wheat kernels, is setting off an aberrant immune response.

Specifically, the gliadin and glutenin are acting as immunogenic anti-nutrients.

Unlike fruits, which are meant to be eaten, grains have a way of fighting back. They create an immunogenic response which increases intestinal permeability, thus triggering systemic inflammation by the immune system—what can lead to any number of autoimmune diseases, including celiac, rheumatoid arthritis, irritable bowel syndrome, and so on. And this holds true for people who don't have celiac disease.

Davis also believes that gliadin degrades to a morphine-like compound after eating, which creates an appetite for more wheat. His claim, therefore, is that wheat actually has an addictive quality to it.

Gliadin, what scientists call the "toxic fraction of gluten," has also been implicated in gut permeability. When someone has an adverse reaction, it is because gliadin cross talks with our cells which causes confusion and a leak in the small intestines. Fasano explains,

"Gliadin is a strange protein that our enzymes can't break down from the amino acids (glutamine and proline) into elements small enough for us to digest. Our enzymes can only break down the gliadin into peptides. Peptides are too large to be absorbed properly through the small intestine. Our intestinal walls or gates, have to separate in order to let the larger peptide through. The immune system then sees the peptide as an enemy and begins to attack.

The difference is that in a normal person, the intestinal walls close back up, the small intestine becomes normal again, and the peptides remain in the intestinal tract and are simply excreted before the immune system notices them. In a person who reacts to gluten, the walls stay open for as long as you are consuming gluten.

How your body reacts (with a gluten sensitivity, wheat allergy or Celiac Disease) depends upon how long the gates stay open, the number of "enemies" let through, and the number of soldiers that our immune system sends to defend our bodies.For someone with Celiac Disease, the soldiers get confused and start shooting at the intestinal walls."

The effects of gluten and gliadin clearly vary from person to person. But as a recent study showed, nearly 1.8 million Americans have celiac disease, and another 1.4 million are likely undiagnosed. And surprisingly, another 1.6 million have adopted a gluten-free diet despite having no diagnosis. In addition, it's estimated that about 18 million Americans have "non-celiac gluten sensitivity," which results in cramps and diarrhea.

Wheat also raises blood sugar. As Davis notes, the glycemic index of wheat is very high... It contains amylopectin A, which is more efficiently converted to blood sugar than just about any other carbohydrate, including table sugar. Consequently, two slices of whole wheat bread increases blood sugar levels higher than eating a single candy bar. Overdoing the wheat, says Davis, can result in "deep visceral fat."

Wheat can also trigger effects that aren't immediately noticeable. Small low-density lipoprotein (LDL) particles form after eating lots of carbohydrates. These are responsible for atherosclerotic plaque, which in turn can trigger heart disease and stroke. And in fact, it has been shown that a wheat-free diet can improve glucose tolerance in individuals with ischaemic heart disease.

Lectins, which are a class of molecules, can be found in beans, cereal grains, nuts, and potatoes. And when consumed in excess, or when not cooked properly, they can be harmful. Now, most lectins are actually quite benign, and in some cases they can even be therapeutic—like fighting some forms of HIV. But the problem with some lectins, like the ones found in whole grains, is that they bind to our insulin receptors and intestinal lining. This increases inflammation and contributes to autoimmune disease and insulin resistance. It also facilitates the symptoms of metabolic syndrome outside of obesity.

Phytates are also a problem, a compound that is found within the hulls of nuts, seeds, and grains. Phytic acid cannot be digested by humans. And worse, it binds to metal ions like calcium, magnesium, zinc, and iron. In turn, these minerals can not be properly absorbed after eating.

Consequently, any minerals that might be provided by consuming grain-based foods are not well metabolized. So phytates, combined with gluten, make it difficult for the body to absorb nutrients—which can lead to anemia and osteoporosis.

Lastly, a common argument in favor of continuing to eat whole grains is that they provide necessary fiber. This is actually a myth. As nutrition expert Mark Sisson has noted, "Apart from maintaining social conventions in certain situations and obtaining cheap sugar calories, there is absolutely no reason to eat grains." And indeed, we can get adequate amounts of insoluble fiber simply by eating plenty of fruits and vegetables.

It is a harsh irony that we have been conditioned to view whole wheat and other cereal grains as not only health foods, but the very foundation of a healthy diet. Even more unfortunately, federal agencies such as the

USDA stand behind the consumption of wheat as if humans never thrived without it.

Unfortunately, cereal grains are a serious concern as both a source of carbohydrates (eaten in excess in the American diet), and as a source of toxic protein compounds. A little-Aknown but important fact is that wheat triggers gut inflammation in nearly everyone. Grain toxins are proteins which are most abundant in the bran, but present in all parts of the kernel. White wheat flour is about 10% protein by weight, while crude wheat bran is about 16% protein by weight. With corn as a close second, wheat is the most toxic of the cereal grains with the following compounds being of most concern (there are certainly others): gluten, a compound protein that triggers autoimmune disease and promotes cancer, heart disease, and neuropathy.

There are also opioids, which make wheat addictive and trigger schizophrenia. Wheat germ agglutinin, a protein that damages the intestine and interferes with vitamin D action (we know that vitamin D is actually a hormone that holds vital importance in the health of the system), thus sabotaging the immune system and promoting chronic infections.

I recommend reading *The Perfect Health Diet* by Paul Jaminet, Ph.D., and Shou-Ching Jaminet, Ph.D. Here is an excerpt from the book that will help explain the toxicity of gluten (and why you should leave bread behind for good):

Gluten is directly toxic to intestinal cells by inhibiting cell proliferation, increasing cellular oxidation products, and changing membrane structure. In the body, gluten changes the structure of the intestine: it reduces the height of villi, decreases the depth of crypts, and decreases enterocyte surface. In other words, gluten sabotages the gut, reduces its surface area, and impairs digestion. Like all toxins, gluten inspires an immune response. This immune response helps to clear the gluten from the intestine, thereby preventing build up of toxins; however, in the process it makes the intestine inflamed. This immune response kills intestinal cells and makes the gut leaky.

There appears to be four levels of immune response to wheat:

- About 83% of the population develops observable gut inflammation after eating wheat gluten.

- About 30% of the population develops anti-wheat-gluten antibodies locally in the intestine.

- About 11% of the population develops systemic antibodies to wheat gluten.

- About 0.4% of the population develops systemic antibodies that attack human cells in the intestine, thyroid, pancreas, and elsewhere.

This last group is diagnosed with the celiac disease. With the immune system attacking and killing gut cells, the intestine can be damaged to the point that sufferers have difficulty absorbing needed nutrients.

Leaky gut is a condition that occurs due to the development of gaps between the cells (enterocytes) that make up the membrane lining the intestinal wall. These tiny gaps allow substances such as undigested food, bacteria and metabolic wastes, that should be confined to the digestive tract, to escape into the bloodstream, hence the term "leaky gut syndrome."

Once the integrity of the intestinal lining is compromised with a flow of toxic substances "leaking out" into the bloodstream, the body experiences significant increases in inflammation. Consequently, the immune system may become confused and begin to attack the body as if it were an enemy (autoimmune diseases). Most often, leaky gut syndrome is associated with inflammatory bowel diseases like Crohn's, and ulcerative colitis, or celiac disease. However, even healthy people can have varying degrees of intestinal permeability leading to a wide variety of health symptoms that can be influenced heavily by the foods one chooses to eat.

Is raw cocoa a superfood or a stimulant?

Even if you've only dipped your toes into the raw food community, you've probably heard tons of raw food gurus promoting cacao as the ultimate tool in the raw food arsenal. But there are others who are vehemently against consuming cacao at all. Who are you supposed to believe? Take a look at this point of view from Diana Stoevelaar, as published on TheRawMan.se in the excerpt below:

Many raw food leaders including Victoria Boutenko, Dr. Doug Graham, Frederic Patenaude, Paul Nissan, Jeremy Safron, Dr. Fred Bisci, and Dr. Brian Clement, have already come to the conclusion that raw cacao is not a superfood but an addictive stimulant.

What do they know that you perhaps don't know yet? They probably have discovered what Dr. Neal Barnard says in his lecture, *Breaking the Food Seduction*. He says that, "Chocolate, just like sugar, elicits an opiate reaction within the brain that trips the dopamine receptors and gives us a pleasure response. I don't mean to say that chocolate is a drug. What I mean to say is that chocolate is the whole darn drugstore!"

When Narcan or Noloxone, the drugs used to block opiate receptors for those suffering a heroine overdose are used in research studies for those with a chocolate addiction, test subjects lose their desire for chocolate.

Jeremy Safron's findings were as follows:

- Cacao is one of the most addictive substances known.
- In some cases of long-term use there are also psychological effects that range from addictive tendencies, sexual dysfunction,

violent outbursts, lack of reasoning, and decreased will.

- At a mega dose of 40 plus beans, it acts as a hallucinogen and can cause many effects that are associatedto LSD or Hashish.
- Cacao is super toxic to the liver.
- The result of long-term use is a high level of liver and blood toxicity, which can cause extreme cases of: mood swings, angry outbursts, violence, depression, paranoia, and dizziness.
- It is extremely clogging due to the toxins carried in the oils contained within. Plus, the fat chains are highly complex and require tons of work to break down.
- It acts as a stimulant and agitates the kidneys and adrenal glands.This can cause insomnia, nightmares, waking up in the middle of the night, shakes, and extreme energy shifts.

- No animal in nature will eat it unless tricked into it with milk or sugar.
- If you can convince an animal to eat it then it greatly shortens their life span if it doesn't kill them immediately (as with dogs).
- The native people who used to eat it only ate the fruit of the theobroma (which contains all the benefits and none of the detriments) and only used the cacao seed as an addition to their psychedelic brew ahyuwascaand as a medicine in emergences.
- Native people did not eat it as a food nor as a supplement, but only for sacred use.

Jeremy Safron's final stand on cacao is that it is for medicinal, sacred and for entertainment usage only. It is not a health food!

Paul Nison says, "The processing of cacao beans into powder and chocolate is an unsanitary, risky procedure to say the least. To be blunt, chocolate and cacao are laced with animal feces and hair, insects, and molds. The carcinogenic mold called aflatoxin has been found in large quantities on cacao beans."

Watch Paul Nison in this very informative 9:33 minute video with references to the scientific research regarding the harmfulness of raw cacao/chocolate:

http://www.youtube.com/watch?v =Jz_XezJ8cMY&feature=related

Doctor Fred Bisci, a raw foodist for about 40 years also confirmed what Jeremy Safron and Paul Nison suspected; Cacao is toxic!!! You can hear him speak about his findings and personal experience with raw chocolate here in this 3-minute clip: http://www.youtube.com/watch?v=-AQA5IJ1oLg

Listen to Dr. Brian Clement explain in this short clip why he does not recommend raw chocolate: http://www.youtube.com/watch?v=GuS WFZO2qso&feature=related

Just last week I was visiting a health food store to purchase my greens (nature's best source of minerals, trace minerals and magnesium) all without stimulants, addictive substances and high amounts of saturated fat, when I got into a conversation with a very health conscious gentleman who asked me what I thought about cacao. I told him that I agreed with Dr. Neil Barnard and others, that chocolate is harmful to our health. Chocolate contains caffeine, theobromine, as well as phenylethylamine, which slows down the breakdown of anandamide just as with the use of marijuana. Now you can understand why it's so addictive!

He relayed an interesting story to me that clearly illustrates raw chocolate's stimulating effects. He told me how he had recently started adding chocolate to his energy sports drink to help his energy and recovery. He rode his bike to the Blood Donor Clinic as he does every two months and tried to donate blood. Unfortunately he couldn't pass the screening test because his heart rate was too high!

They asked him to sit for 15 minutes to allow his heart rate to normalize, but it was still too high. He was shocked since this had never happened to him before! Adding raw cacao was the only thing he had changed in his diet.

Now, you might wonder why chocolate would make his heart race? It's due to the caffeine and theobromine, a sister molecule to caffeine, the same chemical that kills many dogs when they eat chocolate! The adrenal glands rev up metabolism so as to quickly eliminate the offensive substance. This is called stimulated energy, which is always followed by fatigue, and therefore creates a desire for more of the stimulant.

I used to be a chocolate addict myself. I used to eat it every day (and I would prefer really dark chocolate). I loved the taste and the feeling it would give me afterwards. However, after detoxing, and changing my diet, and finally eating fruits and greens, the time came where I had a strange experience with this addictive substance.

At first, I gave up chocolate cold turkey when I learned all the above facts about it and after that, every day, I was craving it insanely. After having it in my diet every day for years, it was something I really needed (at least I strongly felt that way). Very often, I would go to the store, walk through the aisles of raw dark chocolate products, and I would even pick up a couple of products, but then I would stop and remind myself all that we know about this addictive stuff. After remembering how detrimental it is to our health, I would take that chocolate out of my basket.

Yet, one day, after I was abstinent from chocolate for about eight months, I decided to go for it. I bought raw, 80% dark chocolate candy. I was so looking forward to finally enjoying chocolate again, but I was very disappointed. Once I took a bite of it, I felt two different flavors that for some reason were separated from my taste: severe sweetness (from agave), and severe bitterness (from cocoa). It got even worse after I swallowed a bite of it—I still had that severe bitter taste lingering in my mouth. I was shocked. How was I not able to taste that before? Well, once you detox and become a fruitarian, your taste buds become much more refined, so you can taste and pick up even the tiniest flavors, and regular flavors become really strong and sharp.

I didn't enjoy my experience eating this chocolate. It was so horrible that I was trying to change that bitter taste of cocoa in my mouth for the next couple of hours by trying every sweet fruit I would find in my way. But it didn't end there. From that little amount of chocolate that I ingested, I believe I got "poisoned," which seemed totally absurd.

I used to eat this stuff every day. Knowing how badly it affects our liver and kidneys, and the entire system—and provided I didn't eat anything new that day, only greens and fruits—I was 100% sure that my "poisoning" symptoms came from eating that little bit of chocolate.

I spent the next two days in bed recovering from my experience. I had a hard time coming to terms with why my body would suddenly reject chocolate in such a violent way, but then I figured it out.

For example: if you take an alcohol addict, he can drink every day and be just fine. He would even be able to function normally and his tolerance of alcohol would be high, which means he can drink a lot of alcohol without feeling that much intoxication or other obvious effects on his body. But once you put this alcoholic into rehab, and keep him clean from alcohol for a prolonged period of time, his tolerance will be dramatically decreased. Now, if you will re-introduce a small amount of alcohol into his system, he will feel all the ill effects of severe toxicity and intoxication that will be followed by a hangover, especially if he is on a raw vegan diet that is much lighter then SAD (Standard American Diet).

I realized that I had a similar experience with chocolate. From that day of my chocolate poisoning, I never touched this stuff again, nor did I crave that insanely bitter taste. Even more, I am now wondering how people cannot notice that severe bitter taste and flavor. I keep wondering what's so good about it (besides the tons of sugar and milk to coat that bitter flavor). As you go further into detoxing, the more surprised discoveries you will encounter in the explorations of tastes and flavors and ill effects of toxic stuff on your body.

What is nori and seaweed?

It's definitely not vegan, since cyanobacteria or flagellates have always been
classified as simple primitive animal cells. I've
found that the majority of people don't really
understand what algae and other "seaweeds"
really are. There's a huge misunderstanding
among vegatarians and vegans on whether nori
and seaweed are acceptable parts of their
respective diets. Unfortunately, it boils down to
a basic lack of knowledge on this type of
marine life.

Algae and seaweeds are composed of
protists, which are primitive *animal* cells
(flagellates and cyanobacteria). Algae is a
single-cell organism, and seaweeds like kelp
and nori are multi-cellular organisms.
Whether they have one cell or millions, they
are still animal cells.

Seaweeds do not produce oxygen—they
use it. This excerpt from
CitizensForSafeDrinkingWater.org gives a
broader discussion on how seaweeds function:

As with all other animals, these are oxygen consumers (not providers), so they will naturally deplete water of oxygen available to fish and all other sea life when excess blood, body fluids, decomposing animal tissues, and animal wastes allow their "blossom" or "bloom" to occur. This results in them "choking" a river, lake or sea! Their plant-like structuring permits any colony of these organisms to take advantage of the water's layered current differentials. Hence, a continuously renewing food supply is provided to all individuals, but of equal survival value to the organism is its additional incorporation of chloroplast-like organelles. These chloroplast-like organelles in these submerged organisms rarely receive any appreciable sunlight for energy conversion value, but do really serve by its exhibiting of plant-like colors to camouflage the organisms as a plants.

This allows them to avoid being devoured by fish and all sea mammals, all of which are obligate carnivores!

It is important for you to understand that all algae and sea-weeds are also obligated carnivores, which means they are filter-feeding upon bacteria, viruses, amoebas, and all decomposing animal fluids, tissues and waste! They also pick, accumulate and concentrate all the toxins of man, industry, livestock, and runoff in the rivers and oceans. That waste is their food and its collection into themselves is their function.

Another point to consider is that all kinds of seaweeds will produce hormones. Introducing additional hormones into your body can have significant effects (a common theme throughout this book!). In fact, some Olympic athletes have even tested positive for steroids based on supplemental use of algae and seaweed for nutritional purposes.

Seaweeds are designed to filter water and keep the natural environment clean. Don't risk ingesting additional hormones, pollutants, or waste by adding seaweeds into your diet!

A few words about dried

fruits

I always thought that dried fruits are healthy for you. Even if they are higher in sugar then raw fruits, all I would have to do is watch my portions—but otherwise, they are a great part of a healthy diet.

Well, then I learned that any dried food products contain inactive B12 analogues, which compete with true B12 for receptor sites. That means that by eating dried fruits we deplete our system of vitamin B12.

Once I learned this information, I stopped eating any dried fruits whatsoever. It was difficult at first, because I felt like dried bananas were my best desert, and I loved to eat them with my tea. I believed that any dried fruits are a much better choice than cookies or pastries, but once you clean up your diet and have dried fruits as your dessert, then the next logical step would be trying to completely eliminate them from your diet.

The only thing I would allow myself to eat was dehydrated, yet raw vegan banana pancakes for dessert—but I would allow myself only one cheat day like that every month or so.

Ironically, dried seaweeds are often touted as "vegan sources of B12" when that couldn't be further from the case (see the chapter above).

Is nutritional yeast healthy?

The first time I learned about nutritional yeast was when I switched to raw foods, and was exploring different recipes. Nutritional yeast, or *Saccharomyces cerevisiae*, is often used by vegetarians and vegans as a substitute for cheese since it provides a "cheesy" taste to recipes. It also supposedly contains a high source of B-vitamins and protein. I had enjoyed nutritional yeast in many raw vegan menu items, and sprinkled it on all kinds of foods. This stuff is absolutely wonderful and delicious!

However, nutritional yeast, as it turns out, is a deactivated yeast that is cultured in a basis of sugar and beet molasses (by the way, all the beet sugar products in the US is GMO the last time I checked, so look into it yourself to confirm this). While it doesn't have any added monosodium glutamate (or MSG), I found out that ALL inactive yeast products contain free glutamic acid. Glutamic acid is a naturally occurring amino acid and many report similar side effects when consuming MSG as when consuming free glutamic acid.

Gabriel Cousens, M.D., Columbia University medical school graduate, author of *Rainbow Green Live-Food Cuisine* and director of the Tree of Life Rejuvenation Center in Arizona, writes: "One of the main foods to avoid is yeast, baker's yeast, nutritional yeast, and brewer's yeast." It promotes a high level of mycotoxicity (or poisoning of the cells due to fungi). Additional studies have also documented toxic nature of free glutamic acid, as found in nutritional yeast.

David Wolfe also expressed his opinion about nutritional yeast in a negative way. According to him, it may cause all sorts of yeast infections in your body.

Dr. Russell Blaylock, M.D. is a neurosurgeon of great respect and a thorough researcher and author. He has explored, in great depth, the relationship of certain types of brain lesions and their cause, and has discovered a clear link to various food additives, which form or contain "free" glutamic acid. These additives, which are used as "flavor enhancers" or "sugar substitutes," include a host of aliases used by the food industry to disguise their true identity which is MSG (Monosodium Glutamate) or free glutamic acid. Some of these aliases include "autolyzed yeast," "yeast extract," "yeast nutrient," "nutritional yeast," and "yeast food." Dr. Blaylock published his findings in 1997 in his best-selling book, *Excitotoxins: The Taste That Kills.*

Dr. Blaylock revealed his findings that nutritional yeast, like its other yeast cousins, contained "free glutamic acid." The "NON-Active Saccharomyces cerevisiae Nutritional Yeast," as used by many vegetarians, contains free glutamic acid, which is the same neurotoxic compound as monosodium glutamate (MSG). Nutritional yeast is classified as an excitotoxin, a classification of neurotoxic compounds. According to Dr. Blaylock, "Free Glutamic Acid (MSG) literally stimulates neurons to death, causing brain damage to varying degrees." MSG is not added to

Saccharomyces cerevisiae nutritional yeast, but it occurs as a direct result of its growth and processing.

What is "free" glutamic acid? Glutamate is one of the amino acids that make up the building blocks of protein. Glutamate occurs naturally in many plant and animal sources of food. It is also produced in low quantities in our small intestines. This naturally occurring glutamate is bound together by other amino acids that make up proteins. However, when proteins are isolated, texturized, autolyzed, or hydrolyzed, the amino acids are no longer bound together to each other as they are found in nature; instead, they become "free" and turn into "free radicals," causing untold damage within our bodies. Amino acids, as they occur in nature, properly bound to other amino acids, are perfectly healthy and necessary. However, when they become "unbound," improperly linked or "free" by a manmade chemical process, they become damaging free radicals.

Nutritional yeast has vitamins added to it. It is primarily made from pure strains of

Saccharomyces cerevisiae grown on mixtures of cane and beet molasses. According to Red Star, a nutritional yeast manufacturer: "After the fermentation process is completed, 'cream yeast' is heated by means of a heat exchanger and held at pasteurization temperatures for a period long enough to inactivate the yeast." This is when vitamins are added, depending on the type of nutritional yeast that is being crated.

All vitamins that are not in a natural form, inert, and not chelated (like in fruits or veggies), are not bio-available to the human system and are perceived as a toxin. In order to make these vitamins in a powder form or a pill bio-available to the human system, you have to chelate them, and this process brings the price of the vitamins to an extremely expensive cost, measured in hundreds of dollars, which makes it inaccessible for the general public.

So, according to Red Star, the high vitamin content of Nutritional Yeast is actually a result of "vitamins added to meet the requirements of the specific type of nutritional yeast produced." I had always assumed that the high vitamin content of Nutritional Yeast and Vegetarian Support Nutritional Yeast was all naturally occurring. I had naively thought that Nutritional Yeast was so nutritious because it was a type of "special yeast." The truth is, it is grown, fermented, and processed in pretty much the same way as other non-baking yeasts, but with "added vitamins" tossed in to boost its vitamin content—vitamis that are not bio-available to our human system, and are actually toxic.

So, after learning all of the above information about nutritional yeast, I decided that it was clear to me to never touch this stuff again. However, this subject is still found to be controversial for some people that strongly believe that it's good for you to use nutritional yeast. I would not recommend anyone for using this product, but I also encourage you to do your own research about it so you can be really sure about how this stuff affects your body and whether it's wise to use it in your diet.

Is soy a health food?

No doubt you have heard all about why soy is (supposedly) such a powerful health food. But should you really be adding soy into your diet? Dr. Joseph Mercola answers it best in an article titled "The Health Dangers Of Soy," published in the *Huffington Post*:

> If you take the time to look into the actual science, then the answer is no. Thousands of studies link soy to malnutrition, digestive distress, immune system breakdown, thyroid dysfunction, cognitive decline, reproductive disorders and infertility, and in some cases even cancer and heart disease.
>
> One of the primary reasons it would be wise for you to avoid soy is that more than 90 percent of soybeans grown in the United States are genetically modified. Since the introduction of genetically engineered foods in 1996, we've had an

upsurge in low birth weight babies, infertility, and other problems in the U.S., and animal studies have shown devastating effects from genetically engineered soy including allergies, sterility, birth defects, and offspring death rates up to five times higher than normal. Soybean crops are also heavily sprayed on with chemical herbicides, such as glyphosate, which a French team of researchers have found to be carcinogenic.

Soybeans—even organically grown soybeans—naturally contain "antinutrients" such as saponins, soyatoxin, phytates, trypsin inhibitors, goitrogens, and phytoestrogens. Traditional fermentation destroys these antinutrients, which allows your body to enjoy soy's nutritional benefits. However, most Westerners do not consume fermented soy, but rather unfermented soy, mostly in the form of soymilk, tofu,

TVP, and soy infant formula. Unfermented soy has the following 10 adverse affects on your body: [as described by the Weston Price Foundation and Mercola].

1. High Phytic Acid (Phytates): Reduces assimilation of calcium, magnesium, copper, iron, and zinc. Phytic acid in soy is not neutralized by ordinary preparation methods such as soaking, sprouting, and long, slow cooking, but only with long fermentation. High-phytate diets have caused growth problems in children.

2. Trypsin inhibitors: Interferes with protein digestion and may cause pancreatic disorders. In test animals, trypsin inhibitors in soy caused stunted growth.

3. Goitrogens: Potent agents that block your synthesis of thyroid hormones and can cause hypothyroidism and thyroid cancer. In infants, consumption of soy formula has been linked with auto-

immune thyroid disease. Goitrogens interfere with iodine metabolism.

4.   Phytoestrogens/Isoflavones: Plant compounds resembling human estrogen can block your normal estrogen and disrupt endocrine function, causing infertility, and increasing your risk for breast cancer.

Let's back out of the article for a moment to talk about soy phytoestrogens. These potent, antithyroid components cause hypothyroidism and some suggest that they even cause thyroid cancer. Why would a plant have phytoestrogens? It's actually part of their natural survival mechanisms, since phytoestrogens cause damage to any animal that eats them.

According to researchers, phytoestrogens are produced in higher amounts during dry seasons. Animals who eat the plants ingest the phytoestrogens and have a lower reproductive rate. This results in fewer animals to eat the plant, boosting the odds that the plant will survive throughout the dry season. During wet seasons, when plants are undergrowing rapid growth, phytoestrogen production slows down.

Let's go back to the *Huffington Post* article to see five more reasons why you might want to avoid soy:

5. Hemagglutinin: A clot-promoting substance that causes your red blood cells to clump together, making them unable to properly absorb and distribute oxygen to your tissues.

6. Synthetic Vitamin D: Soy foods increase your body's vitamin D requirement, which is why companies add synthetic vitamin D2 to soymilk (a toxic form of vitamin D).

7. Vitamin B12: Soy contains a compound resembling vitamin B12, which can not be used by your body. Therefore, soy foods can actually contribute to B12 deficiency, especially among vegans.

8. Protein Denaturing: Fragile proteins are denatured during high temperature processing to make soy protein into isolated and textured vegetable protein (TVP). Chemical processing of soy protein results in the formation of toxic lysinoalanine and highly carcinogenic nitrosamines.

9. MSG: Free glutamic acid, or MSG, is a potent neurotoxin. MSG is formed during soy food processing, plus additional MSG is often added to mask soy's unpleasant taste.

10. Aluminum and Manganese: Soy foods contain high levels of aluminum, which is toxic to your nervous system and kidneys, and wreaks havoc on your baby's immature metabolic system.

Soy's anti-nutrients are quite potent. Drinking just two glasses of soymilk daily provides enough of these compounds to alter a woman's menstrual cycle.

The Whole Soy Story: The Dark Side of America's Favorite Health Food, by Kaayla T. Daniel, Ph.D. references a study conducted on cheetahs in the Cincinnati Zoo. These cheetahs were not reproducing and had liver disease, both stemming from the soy protein contained in their food. Because they do not have the right liver enzymes to break down phytoestrogens, the cheetahs were especially susceptible to damage caused by ingesting soy.

But cheetahs are not the only animals that can suffer damage from soy. All animals are at risk from ingesting too much soy, with similar effects as synthetic estrogen (often given to animals to stimulate growth). In humans, some studies suggest that soy is a key factor in menstrual issues, infertility, and a range of additional reproductive issues. As Dr. Joseph Mercola explains:

But if you feed soy to your infant or child, these effects are magnified a thousand-fold. Infants fed soy formula may have up to 20,000 times more estrogen circulating through their bodies compared to those fed other formulas. You should NEVER feed your infant a soy-based formula! In fact, infants fed soy formula take in an estimated five birth control pills' worth of estrogen every day.

As dangerous unfermented soy is, fermented soy from organic soybeans is a different story altogether, and can be a beneficial part of your diet. Fermented soy is a great source of vitamin K2, and K2 (combined with vitamin D) is essential in preventing osteoporosis, cardiovascular disease, dementia, and various types of cancer. Note that tofu is NOT fermented. Traditionally fermented soy products include: Miso, Tempeh, Natto, Soy sauce (as long as it's fermented in the traditional way, and if it doesn't contain wheat).

Contrary to what you may have heard, Asians do not consume large amounts of soy. They use small amounts as a condiment (about two teaspoons daily), but not as a primary protein source. And the type of soy they consume is traditionally fermented soy.

The Whole Soy Story provides an in-depth look at the beginning of soy, what it was used for, and how we use it today. Here's an online review from OptimumChoices.com that might prove helpful (and I certainly recommend taking the next step and reading the book):

The Chinese first started eating soybeans about 2,500 years ago, after they figured out how to ferment it. Somehow, the ancient Chinese knew that soybeans still contain many toxins after cooking, and thus, avoided eating it until they learned to neutralize those toxins through fermentation. Soy was originally considered an inedible plant, used to fix nitrogen in the soil. Even today you can find people from farming families who remember that as the primary use of soy.

Soy was also used to lower testosterone levels. Tofu was first used in monasteries in China about 2,000 years ago, in part to promote sexual abstinence, since the phytoestrogens in soy can lower testosterone levels (so maybe there really is something to the saying that "real men don't eat tofu"). Except in times of famine, tofu was only used as a condiment, with pork, seafood and other forms of protein being preferred.

The Japanese probably started eating miso (which is fermented) about 1,500 years ago. Tempeh (another fermented soy food) was not invented until after 1,000 AD when soy came to Indonesia, and it was considered a food for the poor. Most Asians eat only small amounts of fermented soy products (miso, tempeh or soy sauce) as a condiment and the

Japanese typically combine it with fish broth and seaweed that naturally contains iodine, helping offset the thyroid-suppressing effects of soy. Soybean milk was never used historically by Asians to feed their children and soy formula was not invented in China until 1928. The soy milk we drink today is a highly processed food, full of the toxins that naturally occur in soy as well as additives to make it palatable, and not the "health food" it is promoted to be.

In American culture, if you step in any store, you will find almost every product on the shelf has soy in one form or another: soy protein, soy oil, etc. It is put in every possible item of foods as meat substitutes, and none of them are fermented. The best bet would be eliminating soy from your diet entirely. But if you must have it, make sure it's organic and fermented. I also found it strange that organic doesn't necessarily means non-GMO. The product can be GMO, but still grown "organically," so beware of such traps in order to avoid any further health issues.

Is soy lecithin toxic?

The first time I found out about the existence of soy lecithin was when I was making a raw vegan cheesecake and it was one of the ingredients of that cake. It seemed to me that if it was in raw foods' ingredients, it should be safe. But then I did some research, and it totally changed my mind about using this product. Here's an excerpt from an article titled "SOY LECITHIN: It Negatively Affects Your Health and Why You Need to Avoid It" published on PacificHolistic.com:

Soy Lecithin has been lingering around our food supply for over a century. It is an ingredient that is used in literally hundreds of processed foods, and also sold as an "over-the-counter" health food supplement. Scientists claim it benefits our cardiovascular health, metabolism, memory, cognitive function, liver function, and even physical and athletic performance.

However, most people don't realize what soy lecithin actually is, and why the dangers of ingesting this additive far exceed its benefits. Lecithin is an emulsifying substance that is found in the cells of all living organisms. The French scientist Maurice Gobley discovered lecithin in 1805 and named it "lekithos" after the Greek word for "egg yolk." Until it was recovered from the waste products of soybean processing in the 1930s, eggs were the primary source of commercial lecithin.

Today lecithin is the generic name given to a whole class of fat-and-water soluble compounds called phospholipids. Levels of phospholipids in soybean oils range from 1.48% to 3.08%, which is considerably higher than the 0.5% typically found in vegetable oils, but far less than the 30% found in egg yolks.

Soybean lecithin comes from the sludge that is left after crude soy oil goes through a "degumming" process. It is a waste product containing solvents and pesticides and has a consistency ranging from a gummy fluid to a plastic solid. Before being bleached to a more appealing light yellow, the color of lecithin ranges from a dirty tan to reddish brown. The hexane extraction process commonly used in soybean oil manufacture today yields less lecithin than the older ethanol-benzol process, but produces a more marketable lecithin with a better color, reduced odor, and less bitter flavor.

Historian William Shurtleff reports that the expansion of the soybean crushing and soy oil refining industries in Europe, after 1908, led to a problem of disposing the increasing amounts of fermenting, foul-smelling sludge. German companies then decided to vacuum dry the sludge, patent the process, and sell it as "soybean lecithin." Scientists hired to find some use for the substance cooked up more than a thousand new uses by 1939.

Today lecithin is ubiquitous in the processed food supply. It is most commonly used as an emulsifier to keep water and fats from separating in foods such as in margarine, peanut butter, chocolate candies, ice cream, coffee creamers, and infant formulas. Lecithin also helps prevent product spoilage, extending shelf life in the marketplace. In industry kitchens, it is used to improve mixing, speed crystallization, prevent "weeping," and stop spattering, lumping and sticking. Used in cosmetics, lecithin softens the skin and helps other ingredients penetrate the skin barrier. A more water-loving version known as "deoiled lecithin" reduces the time required to shut down and clean the extruders used in the manufacture of

textured vegetable protein and other soy
products.

In theory, lecithin manufacture
eliminates all soy proteins, making it
hypo-allergenic. In reality, minute
amounts of soy protein always remain in
lecithin as well as in soy oil. Three
components of soy protein have been
identified in soy lecithin, including the
Kunitz trypsin inhibitor, which has a
track record of triggering severe allergic
reactions even in the most minuscule
quantities. The presence of lecithin in so
many food and cosmetic products poses a
special danger for people with soy
allergies.

...Lecithin has been touted for years as a
wonder food capable of combating
atherosclerosis, multiple sclerosis, liver
cirrhosis, gallstones, psoriasis, eczema,
scleroderma, anxiety, tremors, and brain
aging. Because it is well known that the

human body uses phospholipids to build strong, flexible cell membranes and to facilitate nerve transmission, health claims have been made for soy lecithin since the 1920s.

Dr. A. A. Horvath, a leading purveyor of soybean health, claims at the time that it could be used in "nerve tonics" or to help alcoholics reduce the effects of intoxication and withdrawal. In 1934, an article entitled "A Comfortable and Spontaneous Cure for the Opium Habit by Means of Lecithin" was written by Chinese researchers and published in an English language medical journal.

Lecithin, though, did not capture the popular imagination until the 1960s and 1970s when the bestselling health authors Adelle Davis, Linda Clark and Mary Ann Crenshaw hyped lecithin in their many books, including *Let's Get Well, Secrets of Health,* and *Beauty and The Natural*

Way to Super Beauty: Featuring the Amazing Lecithin, Apple Cider Vinegar, B-6 and Kelp Diet.

Lecithin did not become a star of the health food circuit by accident. Research took off during the early 1930s, right when lecithin production became commercially viable. In 1939, the American Lecithin Company began sponsoring research studies, and published a 23-page booklet entitled *Soybean Lecithin* in 1944. The company, not coincidentally, introduced a health food cookie with a lecithin filling known as the "Lexo Wafer" and a lecithin/wheat germ supplement called Granulestin.

In the mid 1970s, Natterman, a lecithin marketing company based in Germany, hired scientists at various health clinics to experiment with lecithin and to write scientific articles about it. These "check book" scientists coined the term "essential phospholipids," an inaccurate term since a healthy body can produce its own phospholipids from phosphorous and lipids.

In September 2001, lecithin got a boost when the U.S. Food and Drug Administration (FDA) authorized products containing enough of it to bear labels such as "A good source of choline." Producers of soy lecithin hope to find ways to help the new health claim lift demand for lecithin and increase prices in what has been a soft market. Eggs, milk, and soy products are the leading dietary sources of choline, according to recent research conducted at the University of North Carolina at Chapel Hill and at Duke University.

...One of the biggest problems associated with soy lecithin comes from the origin of the soy itself. The majority of soy sources in the world are now genetically modified

(GM). Researchers have clearly identified GM foods as a threat to the environment, pollution of soils, and a long-term threat to human health with unnatural genetic material that may have unknown long-term consequences with links to decreased fertility, immunological alterations in the gut and the exacerbation and creation of allergies.

Genetically engineered soy contains high concentrations of plant toxicants. The presence of high levels of toxicants in the GM soy represents thousands of plant biochemicals, many of which have been shown to have toxic effects on animals.

The manufacture of soy lecithin is also typically confined to unfermented sources because it is quicker and cheaper to make. Unfermented soy products are rich in enzyme inhibitors. Enzymes such as amylase, lipase, and protease are secreted into the digestive tract to help break down food and free nutrients for assimilation into the body. The high content of enzyme inhibitors in unfermented soybeans interferes with this process and makes carbohydrates and proteins from soybeans impossible to completely digest.

Unfermented soy has been linked to digestive distress, immune system breakdown, PMS, endometriosis, reproductive problems for men and women, allergies, ADD and ADHD, higher risk of heart disease and cancer, malnutrition, and loss of libido. It is now widely recognized that the only soy fit for human consumption is fermented soy.

Similar research has also shown that soy lecithin is being extracted with acetone. Acetone is a nail polish remover—MEGA TOXIC! Besides that, soy lecithin is also way too easy to get: they have it in EVERY health food store, so when something is too easy to get, I can't help but ask questions. Soy lecithin affects and changes our DNA.

After learning all of the above mentioned facts, it is hard to believe that anyone who realizes the dangers of soy lecithin would intentionally buy any product that contains this ingredient. And I know from my own experience; it's not easy to say NO to a wonderful, raw cheesecake. But I learned to look up the ingredients on the cover of the package, and if it had soy lecithin (which I bet most of the "sweet stuff" does—if it's sold in the store, it's got to have it to extend the shelf life), I would just pass on it.

Before I knew how dangerous soy lecithin was, I was indulging in products that contained it, but luckily enough, I found the truth. It is a common mistake that newcomers to the raw foods community make when they start using this product, mistakenly believing it's healthy.

Are beans good for you?

The following information comes from the book *Eating for Beauty,* written by David Wolfe. David, as an experienced raw foodist for decades, shares his knowledge in many books he wrote, and this is one of the books that I highly recommend reading.

The Pythagoreans, like the Egyptians who preceded them, abstained from eating beans. They held beans to be unclean. Beans (legumes) contain coarse, irritating proteins that cause inflammation. Beans naturally contain a host of alkaloid toxins. These protect the beans from animals that would eat them in the wild. Several of these compounds are toxic cyanoges, such as cyanide (found in wild lima beans). Raw beans and peas also contain hemagglutins (causing the blood to clump up) as well as substances that inhibit the digestion of protein. Raw fava beans are very toxic, containing vicine, covicine, and isouramil.

Some individuals cannot break down these toxins at all. These toxins inhibit red blood cells from delivering oxygen to the rest of the body, resulting in headaches, dizziness, nausea, vomiting, severe abdominal pain, and fever. Though these toxins are mostly destroyed by cooking, their presence indicated that beans are not a natural food for human consumption.

Raw peanuts would be the better type of bean to eat (yet are still toxic to our system). Unfortunately, they are typically contaminated with aflatoxin, a harmful fungus.

Soybeans are the least coarse among the beans. They contain more fat relative to protein (but they are still toxic to your body, please refer to the chapter on soy).

However, soy oils (e.g. partially hydrogenated soybean oil) have an anti-thyroid effect that slows down the thyroid, leading to a slower metabolism and weight gain. Eating raw soybeans may enlarge the pancreas, as they contain toxins known to be protein uptake inhibitors.

In my personal experience, whenever I ate beans, I would have a lot of gas and indigestion, so I gave up eating them. Once I have learned that more then 90% of soy beans are GMO in the US, I was avoiding all soy products like fire. And after I learned that you are supposed to eat only fermented organic soy (please refer to the chapter on soy), I realized what a mistake I was making. I would allow myself once in a great while to enjoy tempeh, or natto—but even though I was eating fermented soy, whenever I would try to eat it, my body would still strongly disagree with it. I would feel discomfort each time I ate it, so I finally gave up beans for good.

Potatoes

The following is also an excerpt from *Eating for Beauty* by David Wolfe:

Potatoes are a nightshade-family food. The nightshade family of plants contains various types of toxins. Some nightshade species, such as datura (jumson weed), henbane, and mandrake, may even be deadly if eaten.

Baked potatoes are not only very sugary/starchy and fattening, they also contain the irritating alkaloid toxins solanine and chaconine, which affect the nerves. Solanine is most present in the eyes and sprouted portions of the potato, butis also found in the skin and throughout the root in lighter concentrations.

I personally loved potatoes; they were very hard to give up for me. It's a staple food of any Russian kitchen. There is something comforting about eating hot boiled potatoes with butter, or eating mashed potatoes. When I started transitioning and detoxing, I would "fall off the wagon" here and there and would make a potato for myself—but I would get sleepy and feel heavy afterwards. Once you get clean and stick with raw foods, anything cooked will bring you down. Your body will spend a tremendous amount of energy fighting the toxins from cooked food, trying to digest it. After a few trials of eating cooked potatoes, I gave up on the idea, since it just created too much discomfort and feeling of tiredness.

I realized it wasn't worth it, so I tried my best to let go of my childhood association of well-being with potatoes, when they were served for dinner for my entire family to enjoy. Those were good times, but there was a new and better chapter in my life that was unfolding in front of me to experience.

What is detoxing? What are the symptoms?

Once they clean up their diets, a lot of people start feeling better. But, at some point, they start experiencing some kind of sickness such as flu-like symptoms, or headaches, or nausea, or tiredness, or other physical shortcomings. They immediately assume that they are lacking some kind of nutrient or vitamin in their diet. As a matter of fact, one of my acquaintances tried to become all raw and vegan (meaning only uncooked fruits and veggies), and she felt really sick within the first year. She went to the doctor, and the doctor told her that she is lacking nutrients from animal products, and she had to start eating meat so she could get better and not feel tired.

With everything you have read in the previous chapters, you now know there is no scientific evidence that would support this statement. On the contrary, it was established that animal products are literally lethal to our

344

human system, no exceptions. It won't kill you today; it's an accumulative process that will get you within a few decades. It came to my attention that doctors are not required to take even one nutrition class (at least in the US), and they really don't know all the information I shared with you in this book. They don't know even enough to cover one chapter, because they are taught to suppress the symptoms of the health problems that you have with medication and expensive procedures—not cure the problem itself.

Long story short, at this point we've already established that you don't really need much to have a full spectrum of nutrition, and if you eat 100% raw fruits and veggies, you are more than good on this one. So, then why do people start feeling "sick" at some point of their lifestyle transition? Can it be avoided? What does it have to do with?

The answer is: everyone will go through the stages of detoxing when they improve their diet. Here's what happens: instead of bombarding your system with constantly incoming toxins from breakfast, lunch, and dinner foods, you give a "break" to your body by eating healthy. Before, your body was only able to try to process newly incoming toxins, as they would be so abundant in your system that the body wouldn't be able to take all of them out. So, the body would try to "store" the toxins in your system, like in your joints, or soft tissue like muscles. A large part of toxins would be stored in the gallbladder and liver in a form of gallstones (your body will do its best to encapsulate toxins in those stones). Parasites would have a good opportunity to hide in those stones as well.

But once you are on a clean diet, your body has time to start "unloading" all the storage that was created over the decades of treating your body like a garbage can. It will start trying to dissolve the stones and remove all that entrapped toxins out of your tissue and joints. Once the toxins are released, they have to travel through your blood in your system to exit.

Here is where the problem arises: there is an over-saturation of toxins that was released into your system.You will start feeling "sick" until the toxins exit your system. It might happen on the second week of your new lifestyle, or a year later—it is a different experience for each person, as we all have a totally different combination and amount of toxins entrapped in our bodies.

David Wolfe stated that if you took your blood test and then went 100% raw for a year and took another blood test, you would see much more toxicity in your blood a year later, because your body would be in a full-blown state and process of releasing all that stuff that was put into your system over decades. Your body tries to detox as soon as it sees the opportunity to do so. Once you stop putting food inside your body, the process of detoxing begins. Fruits pose the least obstruction to your system to "clean up the house" and detox. The more complex the meals are, the harder the body has to work dealing with those foods and less energy can be allocated to detoxing.

Personally, when I started a 100% raw diet (of course, I would fall off the wagon every once in a while), I started detoxing big-time. I was releasing so many toxins at once that my immune system couldn't cope with it. I collapsed.

I had a very rocky first year when I went raw. I was sick a lot and I stayed in bed a lot. It was very hard to believe back then that I was "doing good" for myself by making myself sick willingly. My father was insisting me to start eating meat and bread, all animal products, and chicken soup "so I could have enough protein."

After all, he was a doctor. My mother (also being a doctor), also highly doubted my plan. It was extremely hard at times to stand against all my old beliefs (especially under the pressure of my parents, who are doctors and know best). On one hand, after doing all that massive research, and knowing the truth and what happens to your body if you eat animal products, I firmly believed that I could cure everything in my body if I went raw. On the other hand, I had that heavy thought of "Oh, my God, I will become malnourished and even sicker and die if I won't start eating chicken, because my parents are doctors and know better." Those were very controversial times.

At the same time, I was researching cancer patients. It seemed that if a Stage 4 cancer patient went on raw diet, they would either improve or completely cure cancer. But, if they ate meat, they would die quickly without any chance to survive. I chose to stick with my new beliefs, even though they were very shaky, and it was very hard to believe that there is a light at the end of the tunnel when I felt sick not for one week, but for months. I would come down with flu-like symptoms for months. Then I would feel better for a few months, only to crash again. But I had an understanding that my body was unloading a lot of toxins and chemicals out of my system and I had to be patient.

I also noticed some small benefits once I went raw. Within a month, my skin started glowing. After not seeing me for a month, my father Skyped with me and noticed that my skin was fresh and I looked rested (which was funny, because I was exhausted back then having only three hours of sleep for many days in a row). It seemed to me that people around me started to notice that the texture of my skin became more even and glowing. I felt like I needed less sleep.

Within six months of being on a raw food diet, I noticed that I stopped having the "vein" problem. I used to have small capillaries break around my eyes producing those purple tiny veins, which you can find on an aging woman. But, within six months, all veins went away, and I hadn't had any "vein" problems since then.

I also realized for the first time in my life the meaning of the word "being constipated." If you go to the bathroom, it doesn't mean that you are not constipated. Once I went raw, I suddenly started going to the bathroom a lot: three to five times a day, and I would wonder how it was even possible that you poop five times more than you eat. At the beginning of this process, I read, it happens to everyone. Later, once you are stabilized, you start going to the bathroom "normally" again. But what is normal? Apparently, it's when you eat a little but go to the bathroom easily and a lot, and it's formed stool, with no problems. And you feel "light" and good all day long. And you go to the bathroom within an hour after consumption of your meal.

At times I would be so sick from detoxing, that I would stay in bed (for months), and it was devastating. I lost my muscle tone, because I couldn't work out. But I stuck with it. I really believed the data and research I read, and knew that at some point I would get better. I realized that over the course of my entire life (with my parents being doctors who started feeding me allergy pills at the age of four), I probably consumed about 6,000 allergy pills alone. My parents would have an answer to any health problem with a different colored pill.

Right before I went raw, I was taking five pills of Zyrtec a day, and they would not help with my allergies any longer. I had to literally stay indoors when the flowering began each spring. My allergies were unbearable, and I had both seasonal and food allergies. After my detoxing diet, in a matter of couple of years, I didn't have to worry about ANY seasonal allergies. I was able to eat and indulge in foods that I used to be allergic to (for example, citrus).

It was a very rocky road of detoxing, but it was worth it. I am still continuing to detox and improve my health every day, but I am going deeper and deeper every day. They say it takes about seven years to completely change your body (every cell in it is replaced by a new one), so you end up brand-new, in a way: new cells, new body, new bones, new tissues. And detoxing comes and goes in waves—you might feel great at first, then it hits you and you feel sick, then a wave goes by, then you feel great again, and so on. It's constantly intermittent ups and downs with unknown periods of times in between.

Each time, your body takes more and more toxins out of your system and goes in deeper and deeper layers to detox. I noticed that people I keep in touch with, and who have been on a raw diet for a long time, stay and look much younger than their peers who eat cooked foods and animal products. As of right now, I can definitely state that my health improved dramatically, and that I had a long time of downtime of detoxing.

I also had about six months in my second year of detoxing where I had terrible headaches every day for three to four months straight. It is very difficult to function and go to the gym to work out if you have a bad headache every day—and even more challenging when there is nothing you can do to fix it except to wait until whatever is going through your blood is detoxed and exit your system.

But that period of time passed and was replaced by a new wave of feeling better than ever. After each segment of downtime, it seems my body came out stronger and healthier. The farther I went, the more positive results I saw, and the more I believed that it was the right way to go with baby steps forward. With each day you gain very tiny amount of benefits, and it's also an accumulative process. Just like with putting toxic stuff in your system takes years to develop into some kind of disease, the process of detoxing is also slow, and you can see real results over a long stretch of time.

Once you have detoxed and drastically improved your health, you will have forgotten how miserable you were before you started. For example, after I finished my liver and gallbladder cleanse (and had about 2,000 stones expelled out of my gallbladder), a very strange thing happened. My right knee healed—my joint was completely healthy. It was such a gradual accomplishment that I had really forgotten that I even had a knee problem to begin with. Even after a few months of intensive leg workouts, I noticed that I wasn't complaining about my knee anymore.

I had a bad knee since I was six years old. Any physical activity would force me to wrap my knee, otherwise it would be out for weeks and I wouldn't be able to walk. At the age of 18, my knee swelled up so bad and the joint was so sore that I had to go to the doctor, who suggested an injection of steroids to reduce swelling and pain. I had to walk on crutches for six months until my knee was healed. Seven years later, my knee went out of commission again for another six months. My knee was so weak that I couldn't work my legs at the gym.

Doctors told me that I would probably spend my pregnancy (if I ever decided to get pregnant) in a wheelchair due to the weight gain and the problem with my knee. So, it was very strange when suddenly my knee was healed.

After I had enough toxins out of my system, which was about one and a half years into my new lifestyle, my knee miraculously healed. Now I can run and do heavy leg workouts without even wrapping my knee. As I previously mentioned, the longer you stick with detoxing (which might be very unpleasant in itself), the bigger of a believer you will become. You will start noticing the positive results of your body healing, re-building, and rejuvenating. But the question is: is it possible to make it so that you don't have to go through this terrible "detoxing"? Or at least have a "smooth sailing" that would make the journey tolerable?

The answer is, yes. Absolutely! If you don't dive 100% into a raw lifestyle but instead, make little baby steps at a time. It will go very smoothly for you, and your body will detox at much slower rates. Of course, it might take you a decade to see the awesome accumulative effect of super health—but you will get there nonetheless. As a starting point, you can give up all dairy products at first and go that way for six months.

Why six months? They say that it takes about six months for your body to renew all soft, crucial tissues of your body, and for your body to re-adjust to the new changes completely.

In six months, you can then give up all bread, flour, baked goodies, wheat, etc. You can find a replacement for everything (you can make raw bread from flax seeds and fruits and veggies), and can make raw desserts. But stick with no dairy (from previous six months) and no flour, processed, or baked goodies on top of it for the following six months. Within a year, you will have already cleansed your diet from dairy and flour products.

The next step would be giving up all meat, fish, eggs, and butter (all animal products). This might take some time to re-adjust and to plan what to eat instead.

The options are endless, but you have to do your homework and find what will work best for you to substitute and replace all old patterns of eating. Once you go six months with no animal products, your body will thank you for it. This is a slow method of transitioning, but it will give you the comfort of slowly unloading toxins, so you won't "get severely sick" in the process.

The next step would be trying to incorporate as much raw meals into your diet as possible. Try to replace your breakfast with only fruits or a fruit smoothie, and lunch with some kind of oriental stir-fry or something similar. The veggies don't have to be cooked. They can be only warmed up in the sauce and can still stay raw and crunchy. Finally, try to have a large green salad for dinner. Eventually, you will start realizing that you need much less food than you were used to eating. You would get full much faster on raw foods as they are all loaded with nutrients, minerals, vitamins, and enzymes (compared to dead, cooked food that is denatured and there is nothing nutritious left about it—no matter what the doctors will tell you).

Finally, with time, it would be totally natural for you to start eating a lot of green-leafed salads (even with no dressing) and fruits. Eventually, you might find yourself to be a fruitarian by default. You wouldn't strive for it, but your body will sway you that way, because you will feel the greatest benefits from it.

It might take years for you to detox slowly, but what matters is that you are doing something to give your body a chance to heal itself. And if you have an urgency to go faster so you can start enjoying the benefits sooner, then you must prepare for a rocky road as I did.

If you go down that road, within a year or two you will see amazing health improvements and changes. Most importantly, you will test the theory of "enough protein" from plant-based choices, and will realize how much better quality of life you might be living from only changing your diet.

There are also extreme cases that require extreme actions. If you have cancer, then I would say you would just have to dive right into it and detox everything at once. It might involve more than a full raw diet—it's more than likely to involve prolonged fasting to fix the problem fast, followed by a raw diet to help your body become strong again.

And remember, the less obstruction to your body (fruits are the least obstruction to your body), the faster it heals—yet the heavier the detox will be.

The heavier the detox, the more "unpleasant" or "sick" and/or "flu-like symptoms" moments you will experience.

Again, it has to do with your body unloading all old accumulated toxins into your bloodstream to escort them out of your body. Once they are out, you will feel new—but the process of detoxing might be very uncomfortable, and it might last a few days, or a week, or months intermittently. For each person it's different. Some people are more conscious about their food choices throughout their entire life, so they might not have a hard time at all if they would choose to become fruitarians.

I had a really rough journey while detoxing, but I gained a lot of health benefits, and I earned them with really hard work. It takes a lot of discipline and faith to go through such a rough rocky road to complete recovery. Most importantly, please do your homework, learn enough information, and take the time to research the proper way to change your diet. If you want to go vegetarian, vegan, raw foodist, or fruitarian, please research the "proper pyramid" for each type of diet and how to make it right. If you dive into a new lifestyle without a clue of how to balance your diet, it might end up badly.

In fact, if you decided to become vegetarian and stop eating meat and dairy (but indulge yourself in pastas and breads) then your health might be even worse than that of people who eat meat and dairy.

If you choose to try a new lifestyle of eating only raw vegan foods, I highly recommend *The Sunfood Diet Success System* by David Wolfe. This book will explain in detail how to transition, what substitute to use for what, and how to avoid rapid detoxing. This book became my "bible" at the beginning of my journey when I didn't know what to eat. Just one cucumber or tomato wouldn't cut it for me at the beginning, so I had to learn what meals I could make and how to make my diet balanced. In his book, David Wolfe actually teaches what to eat and why and how it will help you with your health. There are awesome recipes in his book as well to get you started.

Gallbladder and liver flush

I don't think I can write and explain better than Andreas Moritz in his book *The Amazing Liver and Gallbladder Flush* about how we get gallstones, how they affect us, and what to do to get rid of them. So, I highly recommend you to invest $20 in this book and read it from start to finish to get a true idea of how our bodies work. Andreas Moritz, an ayurvedic doctor, M.D., cured thousands of his patients only by supervising them in their liver and gallbladder flushes.

In my personal experience, after 12 flushes, I can tell you that it is truly a beneficial experience that helped me cure a lot of ailments that I had since the age of six. I will try to briefly summarize why we get the stones and how to flush them, as well as why it works (there is some really controversial information that Andreas Moritz's method doesn't work and that our body forms those "stones" overnight from the process of ingesting oil mixed with lemon juice, which is not true).

When we consume animal products as well as cooked foods, we acquire a lot of saturated fat and a lot of toxins in our systems. To protect itself, the system tries to "hide" (i.e., encapsulate) the toxic matter and the saturated fat somewhere in the body once it feels that it's overloaded with this stuff and can't get rid of it after ingestion.

Keep in mind that it is an accumulative process of forming stones that happens over months and years, and once they are formed, they grow bigger. Andreas Moritz explains in great detail how the body works on a chemical level, and why it is inevitable that people who consume dairy, animal products, cooked fried foods, and toxic processed foods end up with over 2,000 stones and enlarged livers that are double their normal sizes.

When I read his book, I thought, "Well, that's all cool, but I really don't think I have any stones. NOT ME! After all, I am athletic, and thin, and somewhat active, and I try to stay away from junk foods (back then it meant deep fried foods and processed sugar), so I just can't see myself having any stones."

I thought that eating "healthy" meant staying away from fast foods, and eating chicken and all those lean foods and salads that are called "healthy" cooked food by the mainstream media and society. But I was also told by another experienced person in this area that, based on the facts provided in Andreas Moritz's book, I am congested with stones—which is why I have allergies and joint problems. My right knee joint was always sore since I was six years old, and I couldn't put a lot of strain on it. So in order to do any physical activity, I had to wear a knee wrap for support, and I always had that "bad knee problem" until I finished my cleanse. After my cleanse, my knee problem mysteriously disappeared.

Back then, I wanted to fix my health issues, so I decided to try to do the flush and see what happens. The first couple of flushes were uneventful. I thought it was proof that I didn't have any stones. However, Andreas Moritz stated that if you are really congested, the first couple of flushes could be blanks—but that didn't mean that I didn't have stones at all.

I decided to do another flush. That's where all hell broke loose. I was shooting stones. All sorts of color and size stones were coming out of me: light green, dark green, brown (more aged ones), calcified white, and they were of all sizes from tiny pea size to huge ones—as large as ping pong balls. They were all different sizes, and there were hundreds of them. Some were soft and light green (younger ones) while some were really rock hard, and much darker brown color (older ones). Some stones which I broke open, looked like the inside of the tree stump (you could see the "circles of life" of the stone, as it progressively got bigger and gained layer upon layer of toxic matter wrapping around one another like a snowball). I was able to see the layers of buildup over the years in a lot of stones.

After a few more flushes, I had calcified stones (white on top, and really, really dense). They were pretty big as well. Then, after about six to seven flushes, I had a blank flush again and I happily thought that I was done with my stones. Based on the book, there was still a chance that I was probably still congested, because I felt the pain in the liver area quite a lot that month. It might have been that it was too early to flush, and stones didn't have enough time to move forward. In the book it said that I was supposed to have two blanks in a row in order to assume that I was done with flushing.

So, I decided to keep going with my flushes. At the very end, the last couple of flushes were really "impressive." Three stones that were the size of the table-tennis ball came out of me. I was really impressed, because I didn't experience any pain when the biggest stones were passing. I had felt discomfort at the beginning of my flushes. I believe it was because I didn't know what to expect. I was partly scared of the unknown. I was afraid of pain, as I was not familiar with the process. But the discomfort that I felt at the beginning was not overwhelming, and I didn't feel anything that can really be called "pain."

Rather, it was an annoying feeling of tightness in my gallbladder during the flush, along with some nausea. I realized that I can avoid nausea altogether by simply not eating the day before my flush and the day of the flush itself, and just drink apple juice instead. That totally solved my problem of nausea. In his book, Andreas Moritz doesn't limit your food intake—you just have to be vegan and eat lighter for a few days. From my own experience, that recommendation didn't work for me. I felt much better if I just didn't eat the day before the flush and the day of the flush itself.

The process of flushing is very simple. You drink apple juice for six days: each day, drink one quart of apple juice 30 minutes before your meal, or two hours after your meal. The malic acid in apple juice softens down the stones in your gallbladder and liver, and makes it easier for them to pass. So, for six days, you are basically going about your regular business without any limitations. The only limitation is that you have to stay vegan for that time. That means you have to avoid animal products and dairy, and try to eat a lot of fruits and veggies. Try to include a lot of salads in your diet. You will have to find time off on the sixth evening and on the following morning till noon. That's the only "downtime" that you will need to stay at home, because you will need to be around the bathroom.

On the sixth day, you can have a light breakfast of fruits (I totally skip it and have just some apple juice). You can also have a light lunch like a salad around noon (I skip lunch as well, and just have some more apple juice). At 1 p.m. you have to stop eating. You have to finish drinking your quart of apple juice by 5 p.m. You can drink more juice and water any time you want. And then...the flush begins. You should be at home starting around 6 p.m.

For the next steps, you will need to have Epsom salt (magnesium sulfate), extra virgin unrefined organic olive oil, and freshly squeezed lemon juice. If you are allergic to lemon, you can substitute it with organic (no sugar or other chemicals and/or preservatives added) cranberry juice. In his book, Andreas Moritz gives a list of different options if Epsom salt is a problem, or if apple juice didn't work for you (some people get upset stomachs from drinking so much apple juice). For all my flushes, I used Epsom salt followed by cranberry juice with olive oil.

So, let's start with Epsom salt. Once it's ingested, it relaxes all the bile ducts, and that makes it possible for stones to pass painlessly. Also, Epsom salt will cause the intestines to empty out, which will prepare a clear pathway for stones to move through.

In his book, Andreas also recommends to do an enema before the flush (to clean your colon out). He also recommends to do an enema after the flush, to make sure that all the stones are washed out from the colon. They exit from your gallbladder into your colon, and if some are left stuck in your colon, you might have a bad headache for days until they exit. This is because gallstones are concentrated balls of toxins. If they get stuck in you, your intestines start re-absorbing toxins from those stones back into your system. I personally had that experience when one of the stones got stuck in my intestines for a few hours, and I developed a terrible headache. But, once the stone was out, the headache disappeared as fast as it had appeared.

You should take four tablespoons of Epsom salt and dissolve it in 24 ounces of water (about 710 milliliters). Then, you should split this into four equal shots (doses). The first dose you should take at 6 p.m. on the sixth day. You can still drink plain water as much as you want, as long as it's 30 minutes apart from your doses of Epsom salt. At that time, you might feel like you need to go to the bathroom to empty your intestines.

At 8 p.m., you should take the second dose of your Epsom salt. At that point you will be running to the bathroom a lot with bowel movements. Your intestines will be cleaning themselves out.

At 10 p.m., you will have to take four ounces (about 120 milliliters) of olive oil and mix it with six ounces (about 180 milliliters) of lemon juice (I used cranberry juice instead). Drink the entire glass of mixed oil and juice in one shot. It's not the best or most pleasant feeling when this mixture goes down your throat, but in my experience, if you don't eat for a couple of days and just drink juice, you are hungry enough to actually "enjoy" this oil. It tastes like a salad dressing, and it takes away the hunger. The juice has to be at room temperature; it can't be cold. It is very important to stay away from cold drinks in general.

As soon as you are finished, you have to lay down on your right side (where the liver and gull bladder are). Try to go to sleep. Once you drink oil and juice, you will stop running to the bathroom, but if you ate that day (even light food), you might experience nausea. Andreas Moritz recommends lying on two pillows in an elevated position. You should try not to vomit for at least 30 minutes after you drink that concoction. In my experience, I felt terrible if I ate food the same day or if I ate the day before. But if I didn't eat the day before (or at least the same day of my flush), I didn't experience any nausea whatsoever. There is nothing really scary or painful about this flush—but if you are scared of the unknown, that can make it more discomforting.

I was scared of my first flush; I couldn't sleep through the night. I was feeling some discomfort in my gallbladder, but it was not pain by any means. Once I was familiar with the process, I was able to sleep without any discomfort.

Set your alarm for 6 a.m., and once it goes off in the morning, you should have the third shot of Epsom salt. You should not drink anything with it (I know, it's very bitter), but the best thing you can do is take a small sip of water to chase the bitter taste down.

At 8 a.m., you should take your final shot of Epsom salt. Your flush officially is over. Starting from the early morning (it depends on your individual system), you will feel the urge to run to the bathroom to empty your intestines. At that time, you should really look in the toilet after you are done, and count how many stones you passed and which color they are. You will be running to the bathroom a lot that morning, so make sure you have the entire morning to yourself. There is no pain involved—only the discomfort of running so many times to the bathroom

At 10 a.m., you can have some juice. And at 12 p.m., you can have a light lunch. Usually, around this time, after I would eat some salad, I would stop running to the bathroom. But that wouldn't mean that all of the stones are out. There might be a chance that some stones are stuck in your intestines, so it's a good idea to either do an enema or colonics to avoid any headaches.

Moritz recommends doing flushes once a month and he says that it takes about 12 flushes on average to get rid of all of the stones. He also states that you should stop doing flushes after you have had at least two "blank" flushes, where you don't pass any stones. Also, please keep in mind that you may not pass stones on some flushes, not because you don't have them, or they are all out—but because you might be congested, and it takes time for the stones to move.

In his book, Moritz gives a list of diseases that you can cure yourself from just by getting rid of stones. In his opinion, stones are a concentration of inorganic toxins, saturated fat, and parasites that are hiding in your liver and gallbladder and congest the proper work of bile ducts.

Once these stones are out, you might feel like your joints are mysteriously healed, your arthritis is gone, your allergies are gone, and your inflammations are gone. In his book, he tells a story about one patient who was waiting for a heart transplant, but was running out of time and, unfortunately, he didn't have the replacement in place. As a last resort, that patient came to Andreas asking for help. He just didn't want to die. Andreas told him to do liver flushes along with diet adjustments (vegan). In six months, this patient not only didn't require surgery, but his heart got very healthy. When he went for a check-up, his regular doctor didn't believe his miraculous recovery, but it was a fact. Just remember: we are what we eat.

When I did my own flushes, I though my flushes didn't work because I didn't feel anything. I didn't feel even the slightest of discomforts while I was passing the largest stones I have ever passed. Obviously, I can't post the pictures of all the stones I passed, because I passed over 2,000 stones. To get a better idea and to be able to see the different ages of stones, please refer to Andreas Moritz's book where he explains in detail about all colors and ages of stones supporting it, with illustrations of his own photos.

Now, I would like to address all sorts of rumors that say: You can't flush the stones this way and that the "stones" are simply a formation of olive oil and juice that interact in your body and form "stones" overnight, which you pass the next day.

This is absolutely not true. Firstly, if it were true, then we would have exactly the same result each time. Same stones (same color, texture, and density) each time from ingesting the same amount of olive oil and juice. How can you explain all this stones that are different colors, sizes, and densities? And how can you explain calcification of some of the stones? This process takes more than one night to form. Also, how can you explain "blanks," which are flushes when you don't pass any stones?

When you are done with stones, and they are all flushed out of your system (in my case, it took a little over a year doing it once a month to pass all of them), you won't pass any more stones, provided you are on the right diet that prevents the formation of new ones. Your diet should not involve animal products, dairy, or cooked foods, especially fried foods. But if we assume that our body forms them from olive oil and juice, then why do we eventually stop passing stones altogether?

The only advice I have is to try it yourself. First, do your research, and read *The Amazing Liver and Gallbladder Flush*. Without the proper knowledge of every detail of the process, it would be difficult to go forward with something that you don't have any knowledge about. The more you know, the easier the process of flushing is, because you know what to expect. He does an excellent job of explaining every step in detail. And once you have tried at least five flushes, then you can form your own opinion, because each flush will give you a very small boost to your health. It might be barely noticeable after one and/or each flush, but it is definitely an accumulative process: after the fifth flush I felt a tremendous difference in my health improvement compared to when I started my first flush.

If someone asked me for advice about how to improve their health, I would have one recommendation: "Start with liver flushes—you will really see the difference." Please make sure that you follow all the little details that Andreas Moritz suggests in his book to achieve the best results. I can't write better than him about this subject, so I strongly suggest reading his book before taking action. Don't go off on my short summary—make sure you get the best out of it by doing your homework and fully researching first.

Colonics

I found it useful at some point of my detoxing to use either colonics or just do an enema at home. I remember the first couple of times how much chemicals were washed out of my system, and how much better I felt healthwise.

I also noticed that during my fasting, if I happened to develop a headache, I would do an enema and the headache would mysteriously disappear. I learned this information first from Matt Monarch's video on YouTube.

He says that all problems come from too many toxins in your system. If you unload some of the toxins by a series of colonics to clean out your intestines, your well-being will dramatically improve.

In my experience, it all came true. If you are on a budget, you can do enemas and still get great results. But if you can afford colonics, I would strongly recommend doing at least 10 sessions to achieve your goals. Still, this subject is controversial, as even with colonics you can't clean out all your intestines. You can only make a portion of your large intestine less clogged, but you won't be able to clean out your small intestine this way (colonics doesn't reach that far).

Colonics will break down toxic excrement so that it can no longer harm your body or inhibit assimilation and elimination. Toxins that are built up over a long period are gently removed in a series of treatments. Your colon can begin to operate again as intended. In this sense, a colonic is a rejuvenation treatment.

Exercise the colon muscles. The buildup of toxins weakens the colon and impairs its function. The gentle filling and emptying of the colon improves peristalsis (muscular contraction by which the colon naturally moves material). Colonics is like taking your colon to the gym.

When problematic conditions exist in the colon, they tend to alter its shape, because the colon is a muscle. It will enlarge due to the buildup of toxins which are not being released.

That, in turn, causes more problems. The gentle action of the water, coupled with massage techniques of the colon therapist, help to eliminate bulging pockets of excrement. It also helps to eliminate the narrowed, spastic constrictions in the colon, finally enabling the colon to resume its natural state.

The colon is connected to every system and organ in the body with the help of reflex points. This is why, when the colonic stimulates these points, it results in affecting the corresponding body parts in a beneficial way, creating overall well-being and health in the body.

Water is absorbed into the body through the colon, which increases the volume of blood. The circulation of the blood is increased, resulting in greater bathing of the cells. This dilutes the toxins and flushes them out, relieving toxemia and uremia, while also increasing elimination of both through the kidneys and the skin, as well as the bowels. This all assists the cardiovascular and circulatory systems and makes them more efficient.

Compression of neighboring organs disappears or attenuates when volume reduces in the colon. You can experience a relaxing effect on organs located above the intestines such as the liver, heart, and lungs. Sensation of lightness may also be experienced.

Colonics also reduces pressure in the intra-abdominal area, which improves venous return from lower extremities and pelvic zone. Colonics relaxes pressure on the hips and on the lumbar column and is also beneficial to their mobility. It relaxes abdominal muscles from the action of water temperature and the massage that accompany the colonic. It increases abdominal muscle tone, due to reducing intestinal residues. It stimulates peristaltic action of the intestines, restoring normal muscle tone and ensuring removal of constipation. It potentially corrects intestinal transit problems such as constipation and diarrhea without resorting to prescription drugs.

You will experience a sensation of well-being due to the elimination of mucus, alimentary remainders not digested, gases, and toxic bacteria. You will also notice relief from inflammation and edema as you eliminate irritating substances.

Colonics might also help in expelling parasites due to alternating water temperatures and complementary additives to colonic water such as garlic and other vermifuge (parasite-killing) herbs. It decreases demineralization of the body because it improves metabolism.

It relieves gynecological disorders such as cystitis and dysmenorrhea, due to reduction of a prolapsed intestine. It reduces risk of complications after surgery because it reinforces natural immunity.

We can infer that colonics (colon hydrotherapy) improves functions of the large intestines, lymph, and nervous system because a connection exists between them in the GI tract. Colonics results in weight reduction and it creates an increase in mental capacity and rejuvenation since it decreases the degenerative process, normal or accelerated, by removing toxic substances that affect biological aging. There are so many benefits of doing such a simple procedure that I would definitely recommend you try it yourself and make your own conclusions.

Colosan

Colosan is another way of cleaning your intestines. It might even be considered better than hydrotherapy, because it works on the entire colon, not just on the large intestines as hydrotherapy does. PureBodySolutions.com does a great job of explaining the benefits of Colosan:

An average person is walking around with anywhere from six to twelve pounds of undigested material fermenting in their intestines and colon!

Digestion is a process of oxidation. That is why we give off heat, carbon dioxide, and sulfur dioxide. Just like a car engine, when there is improper oxidation, some of the fuel gets left behind as a residue. There is a similar build up of partially digested gunk in the digestive tract. In an automobile, when you add oxygen to the fuel mixture, the mixed up materials are burned off or oxidized. You can do the same for your body. As these materials accumulate and subsequently begin to rot, your body wraps them in mucus in order to keep them from poisoning you.

Colosan turns the accumulation and the mucus into carbon dioxide and water that are gently eliminated. It is unimaginable to think of going one week without using a toothbrush or toilette tissue. Yet, we forget to clean something important in our body.

When was the last time you thought about cleaning the twenty feet of intestines in between? Do you think it's any cleaner? It's a simple fact, people rarely clean where they can not see and that is where the problems begin.

Your impacted material is home base to four of the most dangerous threats to your health. Number one, it is where the toxins accumulate.

For example when you are behind a bus in traffic, the exhaust gets in your saliva and sinuses. Then you swallow and that chemical soup is absorbed into the impacted material and eventually leaches toxins into your bloodstream.

Second, it is where the bacteria hides when your immune system chases them out of your bloodstream. There they breed and re-infect. Third [and fourth], the impacted material is a fecal fortress for parasites to reside in and an ideal garden for the overgrowth of undesirable flora such as Candida. By using Colosan to oxidize and eliminate this impacted material, you are eradicating the home base to four of the largest assailants to your health and giving them nowhere to hide.

Colosan is also vital to the operation of two very important gut functions—assimilation and elimination. The colon is approximately three to five feet long. The walls of it are reasonably smooth and it is primarily an organ of elimination. If the colon is clogged with mucus and undigested material, the function of elimination is impeded.

Many practitioners recommend health regimens that involve the detoxification of the liver, kidneys, the bloodstream, and the lymph. However, if the colon is not cleaned first, these systems have nowhere to empty and back up. This creates a feeling of malaise known as a detox reaction, or healing crisis. These episodes are unpleasant and can be avoided by using Colosan prior to any detox regimen. By cleaning out the colon with Colosan first, it enables the detoxification regimen to proceed without any impediment and, in fact, can be pursued more aggressively and to better effect.

The intestines are approximately twenty feet long. Nature designed them with a maximum amount of surface area for absorption. The insides of the intestines consists of villi. These are hundreds of finger-like projections making the internal texture of the intestines much similar to a shag rug. When the villi get pasted down with mucus and impacted material, they are less able to absorb nutrients from food or get maximum benefits from your supplementation. Instead, you are reabsorbing toxins from the impacted material as it ferments. By cleaning out the intestines, you enable yourself to get the maximum benefit out of the food that you eat and from the supplements that you take. It is also a wonderful way to reduce bloating and relieve that lousy tired feeling that one gets from absorbing poisons into the bloodstream through the intestines, instead of nutrients.

Colosan is in a powder. It is oxygen and ozone bonded to magnesium. A heaping teaspoon is dissolved in a 12 oz glass of water. A glass of water with dissolved Colosan is followed by the juice of half a lemon, squeezed into the same glass with a dash [of some] more water.

Colosan releases a tremendous amount of oxygen and ozone in the intestines and colon for the purpose of cleansing. Typically, when a person first gets a jar of Colosan, they will take it two or three times a day for a week for an initial cleanse, after which an individual would be inclined to take it once or twice a week for maintenance.

It is important to take Colosan on an empty stomach and wait an hour before eating anything else. The lemon juice assists the hydrochloric acid in your stomach to cause Colosan to release oxygen. This simple reaction allows it to pass into your intestines and colon quickly. There are three times a day when most people find that they have an empty stomach and will not be consuming anything for an hour. These are first thing in the morning, around five o'clock in the afternoon, and right before bed.

Colosan is widely regarded by Practitioners as the most thorough, gentle cleanse that utilizes and complements the body's natural process of oxidative digestion. It is preferred to herbal micro toxins and amphetamines, which purge the body of valuable water...it will help you to empty out undesired materials from your intestines and your colon once they are reduced into carbon dioxide and water.

One can expect copious, aqueous stools but should not experience gas as all reactions take place in solution. This is to be distinguished from diarrhea where by diuretic action or microbial invasion the body purges itself of valuable fluids and there is a sense of urgency. With Colosan, you will have no sense of urgency, which is one more reason why it is the product of choice for colon hygiene. In fact, Colosan is used by many colon hydrotherapists as an adjunct to their colon irrigations or colonics, because it allows them to clean the intestines as well as the colon. With proper colon hygiene health, vitality and longevity can begin in the colon.

Saltwater flushes

A saltwater flush is another way of cleaning the entire GI tract, but unfortunately, it is not for everyone. A small percentage of people are not affected by it and will not flush. I'm not exactly sure why, but it's speculated that it may be a result of sodium deficiency, weakened kidney function, adrenal exhaustion, internal damage to the lining of the GI tract, or a combination of all of the above. I have also found that individuals who tend to retain water (especially women close to their menstrual cycle) do not do well with saltwater flushing. They generally don't flush and retain the salt solution instead. If you have a tendency to retain water, this method is not for you. However, everyone is different and for some it will work, and for some it won't.

Another opinion is that saltwater flushes always work, no matter what, provided you have a strong enough solution (which is slightly different for each person). Still, there is a general rule on the suggested dose to follow. I know people who had to increase the amount of salt in the water in order to have a successful flush.

A saltwater flush is an effective tool to help keep your colon healthy and clean. What's even better is that it acts as a mop for your entire GI tract, sopping up everything from top to bottom. It can help with digestive irritablility, gas, bloating, cramping, etc.

Usually it is recommended to do the flushes daily for a week, and then once a week for maintenance. You should drink a saltwater flush solution first thing in the morning. It requires high-quality, untreated salt and a large volume of water. The salt water's saliency is the same as the body's saliency. So, hypothetically, none of the water gets absorbed into the body. It just passes right through you and out through your colon. Therefore, it simply makes its way through your GI tract causing a "tidal wave" effect, pushing everything along until it comes out the other end.

<u>Instructions on how to use it:</u>

1. Use only unrefined and unprocessed Premium Himalayan pink salt. This is the best choice for the flush.

2. Saltwater solution is used as the first thing in the morning before any food and drink.

3. Add one heaping tablespoon of Himalayan salt to one quart of room-temperature, filtered or RO water.

4. Try to drink the entire salt solution within 15-20 minutes. Some people can do it within five minutes. Drink another half to one quart of pure water within an hour after taking the salt solution. Don't eat for at least a few hours and avoid coffee, tea, or anything that may be dehydrating. It is best to stick with water.

I read that some people recommend to lay down after drinking saltwater while others recommend to move around to help the water go through your intestines. Also, some suggest to drink not one but two quarts of this salted solution in one take (and yes, in each quart you have to use one heaping tablespoon of Himalayan salt).

Most people experience several bowel eliminations within one to two hours of intake. You will need to visit the bathroom frequently, so plan accordingly. You are generally safe to leave the house within a few hours. If the last bowel movement was mainly clear fluid, then this is an indication that you have completely flushed your GI tract. For some individuals, this may not happen at first. They may have several eliminations but not a complete GI flush. It may take a few saltwater flushes to accomplish this.

I don't really have a personal opinion on saltwater flushes, because I don't have much experience in this area. But I have heard so many good things about it that I decided that it might be an important tool for you to choose from among the variety of methods of how to start cleaning your GI tract.

Golden Coin Grass (GCG)

This tincture is traditionally used for softening and crushing gallstones, as well as preventing kidney stones and gallstones. It is often used to prepare for a liver/gallbladder flush, to alleviate gallstone-related pain by softening and crushing the gallstones. GCG affects the liver, gallbladder, kidneys, and urinary bladder. It is very easy to use. You need to take one tablespoon (about 15 mL) once, daily on an empty stomach, 20 to 30 minutes before breakfast.

The secondary ingredient of GCG is Bupleurum, also known as Chai Hu or Bupleuri Radix. The literal English translation of the name is "Twigs of the Barbarians." According to medical research, this herb may stimulate immune system function. In Chinese medicine, it is considered as a "cooling" herb and is used to treat flu and fever. It is also said to decongest the liver, so it is often used to treat women's problems such as irregular menstruation.

I used GCG before each liver and gallbladder flush I did, and I had wonderful results. GCG helped to crush my stones in the gallbladder and during the flush, I saw broken fragments of larger stones come out instead of full stones. When I was taking GCG (for a duration of one week, before I did the flush by Andreas Moritz—please see the chapter on liver and gallbladder flush), I felt my gallbladder moving and tightening throughout the day, almost like contractions that helped the stones get crushed inside. I can totally support the claims that GCG is a miraculous supplement.

I initially started taking GCG because my fourth flush was a blank and I figured I was likely very congested and stones were too large and couldn't pass, so I took GCG. Sure enough, during the next flush I passed a lot of crushed stones. You can find this product online. I haven't seen it at the stores, but it is really easy to Google it and it's fairly inexpensive. It only costs $20 or so and it will last two to three weeks, so you can use it for two or three liver and gallbladder flushes.

Chanca Piedra

(Stonebreaker)

"Phyllanthus niruri" is the latin name of this wonder plant, famous in America as Chanca Piedra (literal translation from Spanish: "stonebreaker"). India is the biggest consumer of this herb as Ayurveda. The traditional healthcare system of India uses this herb formally in its medical health care. There are also many doctors who recommend this herb and formulations made from this herb for Liver cirrhosis, Ascites, stones, and Hepatitis. That is why this herb is also called stonebreaker. The herb is described in almost all the books of ancient Ayurvedic medicine.

"Phyllanthus niruri" has been proven in over 80 clinical and laboratory studies to have the following medical benefits:

- **Smooth muscle relaxant** – In particular the stomach, ureter, bladder, and uterus, which is why it should not be used by pregnant women

- **Antilithic** – Dissolves calcium crystals that are responsible for the formation of kidney stones and prevents the formation of new stones
- **Hepatoprotective** – Helps heal and protect damaged livers
- **Antiviral** – Shows positive effect against HIV and hepatitis B and C
- **Analgesic** – Shown to be a highly effective pain killer for certain types of pain, in particular the types of pain experienced by kidney stone sufferers and post-operative pain
- **Hypocholesterolemic** – It lowers LDL (bad) cholesterol and increases HDL (good) cholesterol,
- **Hypoglycemic** – Naturally lowers blood sugar to within normal ranges

- **Hypotensive** – Naturally lowers blood pressure
- **Antispasmodic** – Reduces spasms of smooth muscle, in particular the type responsible for kidney stone pain
- Antimutagenic – Inhibits the growth of certain types of cancer cells, in particular sarcoma, carcinoma, and lymphoma

"Phyllanthus niruri" dissolves and eliminates gallstones, prevents new gallstone formation, and is high in antioxidants and phytonutrients.

Speaking from my friend's experience, it really works. She had kidney stones, which she found out by getting an ultrasound. She went and bought Chanca Piedra (it cost around $15.00 dollars) tincture and started taking it twice a day—one full dropper at a time. Within six months, all her stones were dissolved (another ultrasound confirmed that she had no stones anymore).

Chanca Piedra dissolves calcium crystals that are responsible for the formation of kidney stones and prevents the formation of new stones. I would suggest taking it for at least six months. As a result, all your stones will slowly disappear from your system. Of course, you should also adjust your diet from an All-American cooked diet (SAD: Standard American Diet) to a raw vegan diet, in order to stop the vicious cycle of formations of the new stones.

My mother was taking Chanca Piedra for a solid eight months to detox and break up all the stones that had built up in her system. She felt like it was non-invasive and a very smooth way of getting rid of stones for her instead of liver and gallbladder flushes, which might seem more harsh to some (although for me, liver and gallbladder flushes were, without a doubt, life-changing).

Dry fasting

Dry fasting has likely been a regular part of many cultures and religious traditions across the span of human history. What is dry fasting? As Esmée La Fleur describes in an article titled "An Introduction to Dry Fasting":

> A dry fast is an absolute, true fast in which you abstain from both food and water. Based on available literature, this is the type of fast that was practiced by Moses (Exodus 34:28 & Deuteronomy 9:18, both times for 40 days), Ezra (Ezra 10:6, length undisclosed), the Nation of Israel (Esther 4:16, 3 days), Elijah (1 Kings 19:18, 40 days), the Ninevites and their animals (Jonah 3:7-10), most likely Jonah himself when he spent 3 days in the belly of the whale (Jonah 1:17), the Apostle Paul (Acts: 9:9, 3 days), and Jesus Christ (Matt 4:2, 40 days).

...In a dry fast, the body eliminates toxins in a similar manner as it does during a water fast. However, each day of a dry fast is said to be equivalent to 3 days of water fast in terms of detoxification, so you accomplish much more in a shorter time.

...The good thing about this is that a person does not need to take a long absence from their normal life, so it costs less both for the fast itself (if you are going to a facility to be supervised) and for the time taken off from work. Also, you lose less muscle mass and more body fat with dry fasting, than you do with water fasting, and the recovery time is quicker. Returning to normal function after a 10 day dry fast is much faster than after a 30 day water fast.

Dr. Filonov is a Russian doctor who has been practicing dry fasting over few decades and cured thousands of people at his facility. In his experience, he has seen many illnesses heal

through dry fasting. Below is a list of the ones
he mentions in his book, *Dry Medical Fasting:
Myths and Reality*:

Ovarian cysts, uterine fibroids,
endometriosis, infertility, mastitis, hot
flashes, yeast infection, parasite infection,
viral infection, bacterial infection, benign
tumors, rheumatoid arthritis,
osteoarthritis, ankylosing spondylitis,
asthma, chronic pneumonia, pulmonary
sarcoidosis, atherosclerosis,
hypertension, sciatica, herniated disk,
brain injury, migraine headaches,
gastritis, stomach ulcer, duodenal ulcer,
pancreatitis, cholecystitis, ulcerative
colitis, irritable bowel syndrome,
hemorrhoids, non-insulin dependent
diabetes, gangrene, atopic dermatitis,
chronic urticaria, eczema, psoriasis,
interstitial cystitis, chronic
pyelonephritis, prostatitis, prostate
adenoma, and inflammation.

Dry fasting has been practiced by the Russians for a very long time. There is quite a bit of literature available on dry fasting in the Russian language. However, none of these findings have been professionally translated.

I was introduced to dry fasting by Akahi and Camila when I did a breatharian retreat with them. They are breatharians, or people that don't require food or water to sustain their lives. In their case, they choose to drink something for flavor once in a great while. During that retreat, we abstained from food for eight days, and within that time period, we went with no water for three days.

This experience was very powerful. Before the retreat, I was very sick and couldn't recover from my ailments. But after three days of no food and no water, I miraculously got back on my feet within a week. It shocked and surprised me at the same time, so I started researching dry fasting and came across Dr. Sergei Filonov, a Russian medical doctor who has been conducting dry fasts with his patients for 20 years.

I got in touch with him and Skyped with him a few times to find out all the details about his experience and knowledge in this domain. It became obvious to me that people can cure stage four cancer within eleven days of dry fasting (some might need two to three repeated 11-day dry fasts with re-feeding in between to achieve 100% recovery). Most parasites die in your system on the sixth and seventh day of no food and no water. Your system gets detoxed very quickly. I read all of Filonov's books, and his insights were extremely educating. I'll provide an overview of his research here for you to begin your own research.

There are two kinds of dry fasts: hard and soft. In a hard dry fast, the person does not allow any water to touch their body (i.e. no washing dishes, no taking baths or showers, no brushing teeth, etc.). With a softer dry fast, the faster can allow their body to come in contact with water.

When you go on a dry fast, the pores of your skin develop a greater capacity to absorb water through the skin and will readily absorb moisture from the air. It is for this reason that Dr. Filonov highly recommends undertaking a long dry fast in the mountains where the air is fresh, moist, and pure. He encourages many of his patients to sleep outside, next to a stream of running water during their long dry fasts.

While several of our Biblical forefathers fasted for 40 days, the longest dry fast on record (again, on record, but not in real life) in modern times is of 18 days. However, most modern practitioners of dry fasting do not recommend dry fasting for longer than 12 days. Dr. Filonov always recommends doing several water fasts before ever attempting a dry fast. Then, he recommends that a person start with very short dry fasts of 36 hours, once a week. After doing this for a while, a person can gradually do longer dry fasts of two, three, and four days. Finally, to affect deep cleansing of the tissues and healing of serious chronic illnesses, he recommends a protocol known as a "fractionated" dry fasting in which the person does a dry fast for five to seven days, re-hydrates for three days, then does a second dry fast for nine to 11 days. He has found this method to be extremely safe.

In order to achieve permanent healing results, a person must traverse two separate "acidotic" crises, the first between three to five days and the second between nine to 11 days. So, by breaking up the fast, the "fractionated" method allows the person to go through the first crisis during the first fast and the second crisis during the second fast, thus reducing the stress on the body from too many toxins needing to be eliminated at one time.

It should be noted that Dr. Filonov never recommends doing a dry fast for longer than five days without supervision. The problem with this is that there are no medical doctors with experience in dry fasting in the United States. We are pretty much on our own if we want to use this method of healing. I also noticed that even doctors that have their own clinics that claim to specialize in water fasting don't recognize dry fasting whatsoever, because they don't know anything about it and are not familiar with the subject.

Another method of dry fasting that Dr. Filonov has found to be extremely safe and beneficial is a protocol he calls "cascade" dry fasting, in which the person begins by fasting one day and eating one day alternately. Then, the person fasts two days and eats two days alternately; fasts three days and eats three days alternately; fasts four days and eats four days alternately; and then fasts five days and eats five days alternately. With this protocol, the person is literally fasting one half of every month. In his book, Dr. Filonov says that he personally knows a medical doctor who cured himself of blood cancer by doing 5/5 protocol for a full year.

Basically, the idea is that one day of dry fasting is much more powerful than water fasting. As a matter of fact, one day of dry fasting is equivalent to three days of water fasting. But it might not be a very "smooth ride" for majority of people. I would not recommend doing any kind of dry fasting without proper supervision until you have enough experience and can do it in the comfort of your home by yourself. I would say three-day dry fasting is very powerful and is totally safe to do at home (but again, you should see professional advice and supervision of someone like Dr. Filonov in order to have a successful journey of fast detoxing).

There is also some preparation time involved. I would recommend to be on raw vegan foods for at least a few months before you try to attempt your dry fasting. I would also recommend to lead into it with a two-day lead-in. You should only eat high water content fruits on the first day—and eat mono-fruits, meaning only one kind of fruit at a time—and then take a couple of hours of a break before starting a new kind of fruit. On the second day, you should only drink diluted juices such as freshly squeezed fruit juices (again, pick one type of fruit, don't mix it). Only then I would recommend going into your dry fast on the third day.

Dry fasting in itself is not difficult and the first day is usually not different from any other day. You can easily go about your business. You might feel a little tired, but it seems like that the first day doesn't affect the person that much. My mother started dry fasting one day a week, and she goes to work and cooks for her grandchildren (my sister's kids) and does all her normal chores, and she feels just fine (and she is in her 70s).

On the second day of dry fasting, however, you should stay at home. The second day is when you will start feeling dizzy and might start having nausea, diarrhea, or upset stomach, or headache. It's different for each person; it all depends on how toxic an individual is. You should be very careful when you get out of bed as blood pressure drops dramatically, and you might black out if you move too fast while changing elevation. I used to walk down the stairs holding the wall at the beginning when I just started fasting. But after over 10 dry fasts, I was able to go about my day and even drive on the second day of my dry fasting. It is ok to have really yellow (even brown) and highly scented urine. You won't urinate that much, but you will still urinate.

Usually, if you dry fast long enough, it clears out—but it might not in a short fast of three days.

On the third day, you will be extremely thirsty. You might be dreaming about drinking. You will literally be counting hours when you can start drinking again. It is a challenge, but it's really rewarding to go all 72 hours before breaking the fast. Also, keep in mind that 80% of your success depends on the time when you are coming out of the dry fasting. It should be twice longer than the fasting itself.

Imagine that you are a "wrung out" sponge, and now you can put in clean water in it to soak all it needs. It's very important to go at least six days after a three-day dry fast on a very clean diet, so all the nutrients you put in your body would be healthy and non-toxic. Otherwise, all your work would be for nothing. Your body, like a sponge, will soak in everything you put in—and if it's not organic and clean, but processed and cooked foods, then why fast in the first place if you won't reap the benefits for your hard work?

Also, it is very important to know how to lead out of the fasting, because if you have cooked lunch or breakfast right after your dry fast, you might end up in the hospital in a very critical condition (especially in fasts that are longer than three days).

It is very important to take this very seriously, and slowly lead out of the dry fasting. I would recommend drinking a glass of water and starting out this way. That is the best way to break your dry fast. If you feel nausea, take your time and take very small sips of water for 15-20 minutes to finish your first glass of water. If everything is ok, in an hour or so, you can put 10% of freshly squeezed watermelon juice in the next glass of water or 10% coconut water (it's very hydrating and high on electrolytes, so it's good to dilute it, especially for longer than three-day fasts to avoid migraines and other unpleasant "surprises").

If that went well, then you can drink juices (one kind at a time). The best juice that would be super hydrating is coconut water (from green coconut, not canned or from concentrate). Only the following day would I would recommend eating high water content fruits (one type at a time), and then sticking to a raw vegan diet for at least six days after you have finished your dry fasting.

I would also recommend staying away from any type of salt for at least a week or more if you can. Your body is clean, and you might swell up a lot (you may even see swelling the next day when you wake up) from eating salt right away. Besides, it would be really counterproductive to ruin all your hard work of dry fasting in order to detox only to ruin it with salt. Salt is non-organic and not bio-available matter that is toxic to our body. The same goes for refined sugar. Nothing processed, baked, or cooked should go into your system at least for the first couple of weeks after you are done with fasting.

What does dry fasting do? It basically cures any and all inflammations you have. No water equals no inflammation. Also, even though you think you are thirsty, your body is not. It digs deep within itself, finds all the "retired" cells—cells that don't function properly, old cells, and toxic and deformed cells, and takes them apart. The toxins from that dead cell are released and incinerated, and liquids and other contents from that cell are used for food and water for your body. You are essentially "unloading" all of the garbage and unnecessary material that was taking your energy, but was not paying off by functioning properly.

I personally did over 30 dry fasts within a year after I was introduced to it. I would go mostly three to four days at a time. But there were cases where I would go three days, then would do a one-day break and try coconut water first, then I would realize that it didn't feel good, so I would go back to dry fasting for another four days.

When I got braver (after over 10 dry fasts) and had much more experience, I went five days, and it took me two weeks to recover from it to be as strong at the gym as before my fast. Also, after that fast, I was not able to use any salt in my food (even if I wanted to enjoy the flavor) as I would instantly get migraines and would swell up a lot the next day.

Salt is very toxic to our body and it is dangerous to start eating it right after you come out of fasting. If you really feel like still keeping salt in your diet, my recommendatios is that you should wait for a few weeks after your fast, and very slowly re-introduce it in your diet. If you think you need salt in your body right away, then do it in organic and bio-available ways, such as celery juice, and you will get all the salts you need.

The longest I went dry fasting is nine days, and it was extremely difficult. I was in bed all the time and it didn't feel great at all. It definitely was the hardest challenge of my life. I felt weak and dizzy. I had a hard time getting out of bed to go to the bathroom. I felt like I would black out if I changed elevation quickly. I also felt nausea and headaches. It wasn't a fun journey, but it felt awesome afterwards when I realized that my allergies were almost non-existent. Dry fasting sure does help with a lot of health problems, and it certainly worked for me.

I would not advise anyone to try dry fasting for the first time at home by themselves. This should be done under someone's supervision (i.e., someone that has good experience and can guide you through it).

I learned a lot before I started doing fasts at home by myself and feel comfortable. I even did one very long fast while traveling cross-country (seven days of dry fasting followed by seven days of water fasting). It was easy, because I traveled by car and was not the driver. So I just got to sit in the passenger seat and enjoy the ride while exploring different destinations. It was a little bit of a challenge to watch my companion eat (for example, the smell of a banana would fill up the entire car when he was eating it), but I persevered.

I was strong, and later on our trip, I switched to water fasting from dry fasting. While I was water fasting, my companion wanted to go to a restaurant and get lunch. So, I would go with him, sit there, and watch him eat his fresh, raw salad while I was drinking hot water (without a tea bag). Usually, after a week of no food, the wish to eat falls off by itself (at least with me), and I am totally fine with being around people eating food. It doesn't urge me to run for my own plate.

Actually, as my experience with fasting progressed, I noticed that the food didn't bother me even on the second day of my fasts. I was able to be around foods without issue. I was even able to cook food for friends while fasting, but didn't feel the urge to eat it. But this was only after I had gained a good foundation of experience in fasting. For now, as you begin your own dry fasting journey, I would recommend you to try small baby steps (like my mother did) and do one day of dry fasting and see how it feels to go without food or water for the entire day.

One day is absolutely safe and fun to do, provided you follow all the rules of proper leading in and leading out. It is of most importantce, even if you do only one day of dry fasting, to make a habit of practicing proper lead-ins and lead-outs. In the future, when you start doing longer dry fasts, you will be safe while enjoying them, because you already will have a habit of proper lead-ins and lead-outs. In this case, you will ensure that you are not endangering your health and are staying safe.

Your weight: The body is not going to build on rotten flesh

It is interesting to address the problem of weight, as some people are afraid of losing too much weight or becoming too skinny. Of course, for those who have a lot of extra pounds to lose, changing your diet is a great way to do it. With each step you take to reach your optimal health, your weight is going to melt away without you noticing it.

Personally, I would recommend a raw vegan lifestyle (notice that I'm calling it a lifestyle, not a diet). It is fun, because while trying out new raw vegan recipes and flavors, your body is detoxing, and you will reach the goal of optimal health effortlessly.

So, how is it that some people might lose weight, but others won't? Why can some people go on just juice, or water, or just an apple a day and still sustain the same weight? And why do some people keep losing weight?

The answer is very simple: if you are acidic, you will be losing weight until your body can clean itself up from the inside out and become alkaline. Once you are alkaline, you will not lose weight even if you are just on water.

Johanna Brandt, in her book *The Grape Cure,* proved this theory time after time. She had cancer patients whom she would put on a grape diet for a few months. At first, the patient would keep losing weight and become literally anorexic—but within a couple of weeks of being in that state, the same patient would start putting weight back on, even while being on the same diet that made them lose all that weight. The difference is that the person would recover completely from a deadly disease and become healthy on a diet of only grapes within few months.

One more interesting fact is that you will be losing weight if you have parasites in your gut. You might never see them (round worms are usually in small upper intestines, so you have no idea that you have them). But parasites will only be in a toxic, congested body. They are your "friends" because they are trying to clean up the mess you made in your intestines. However, they also release excrement, which is toxic for us.

Once your intestines are clean of all that trash and all that plaque (which is stuck to the walls), they will either starve to death and die or exit your system on their own. Parasites (including fungus) will be found only in acidic bodies. Once the body is clean and alkaline, parasites won't be able to survive in those conditions.

Basically, the body won't build up on rotten and sick and toxic matter. It will "clean the house," deconstruct, and then reconstruct. It takes a lot of discipline, patience, and the right guidance to believe in it and go through with it.

After my last fast, which was about 35 days of a water fast, I went from 105 lbs to 74 lbs. I looked anorexic. I was extremely weak, and it was a great achievement for me to get out of bed and walk to the bathroom. I was not even able to hold my own weight. It took me 2.5 months to put 20 pounds back on, just by eating watermelons. Yes, that's right, I was only eating watermelons—and it worked (I was under supervision of an experienced person). I was very patient and it took a lot of time to see those small gains. But the basic idea is that if you are not acidic, you are super healthy and that means you are alkaline.

If you are alkaline, you will not lose weight, even if you are just drinking water. If you are acidic, you will be losing weight until your body completely cleans itself and detoxes, before it turns around and you start gaining weight back.

Superfoods: Goji Berries, Camu Camu, Maca, Shilajit

I would like to mention a few super foods that I used when I started on a raw vegan diet. I found these four superfoods very useful to me, so I think it might be interesting for you to learn something that could be quite helpful (especially if it isn't widely advertised yet).

Goji berries

Goji berries (Lycium barbarum) are the most nutritionally dense fruit on Earth. They are a member of the nightshade family (Solonaceae), which contains many other common vegetables such as potato, sweet potato, tomato, eggplant, and pepper, as well as some poisonous plants like belladonna and deadly nightshade. Native to the Himalayan Mountains of Tibet and Mongolia, the goji berry is now grown in many other countries as well. Although they have only recently been introduced in Western countries, gojis have been used for thousands of years in Tibet and China, both as a culinary ingredient and medicinally. This is the only known fruit that naturally stimulates the production of HGH (human growth hormone), which might be the reason why people that consume it on a regular basis, gain much higher longevity time span and live a way over 100 years.

Unique among fruits because they contain all the essential amino acids, goji berries also have the highest concentration of protein thenany other fruit. They are also loaded with vitamin C, contain more carotenoids than any other food, have 21 trace minerals, and are high in fiber. Boasting 15 times the amount of iron found in spinach, as well as calcium, zinc, selenium, and many other important trace minerals, there is no doubt that the goji berry is a nutritional powerhouse.

This amazing little superfruit also contains natural anti-inflammatory, anti-bacterial, and anti-fungal compounds. Their powerful antioxidant properties and polysaccharides help to boost the immune system. It's no wonder then, that in traditional Chinese medicine they are renowned for increasing strength and longevity.

In traditional Chinese medicine, the goji berry is said to act on the kidney and liver meridians to help with lower back pain, dizziness and eyesight.

Gojis are most commonly available in dried form, and make a great snack eaten as is. They can also be soaked for a couple of hours in enough water to cover them. Then the soaked water can be drained off and it makes a delicious drink, or both water and berries added to smoothies.

Please note that there can be some adverse interactions if you consume goji berries while also taking medication for diabetes or blood pressure, or you take the blood thinner *Warfarin*. So, be sure to consult your health care provider.

Gojis can often be found in Asian food stores, but most of these come from the commercial growing regions of China and Tibet and contain high levels of pesticides and synthetic fertilizers. Even some brands, which claim to be organic may not actually be, so be sure to source your goji berries from a reputable source.

Camu Camu

This isn't a fruit you'll find on a tree or bush in your neighborhood. I've paraphrased an article titled "Camu Camu Benefits: 11 Things You Need To Know About The Fruit" written by Terri Coles in the *Huffington Post* for you below:

Camu camu mostly grows in the flooded areas of the Amazon rainforest in Peru, Brazil, Colombia, and Venezuela, where its fruits and leaves are used for medicinal purposes. Its fruits are about the same size as a lemon, but it is light orange in color and is full of vitamin C.

Some claim that camu camu has anti-viral properties that can help with cold sores, herpes, shingles, and the common cold. Others say it's a natural energy booster that's great for your eyes and gums. Here are the benefits of camu camu:

1) Camu camu is full of vitamin C: 60 times more per serving than an orange! A teaspoon of camu camu powder has 1180% of your recommended daily intake for vitamin C, which is important for gum health, among other functions of our body. [Also, it might help with allergies, as vitamin C is anti-histamine.]

2) Valine is an amino acid found in camu camu. It is an essential amino acid, meaning that we must get it in food because our bodies cannot produce it [at least, so they say]. Valine is used by the body to prevent muscle breakdown and is important for nervous system and cognitive function.

3) Our bodies need potassium for the proper functioning of the heart and kidneys. Camu camu is one way to get it: 71.1 milligrams are found in every 100 grams.

4) Leucine is another essential amino acid found in camu camu, one that our bodies need for muscle and bone tissue growth and recovery and for the production of growth hormones.

5) Serine is another amino acid that is key for digestion. Serine helps to break down the bonds in proteins and polypeptides, so they can be used by our bodies.

6) Camu camu has several different flavonoids, which are compounds that are found in plants and are part of what gives fruits and vegetables their awesome colors. They mostly function in the body as antioxidants, neutralizing harmful free radicals.

7) Gallic acid is also found in camu camu, which appears to have anti-fungal and anti-viral properties. It also acts as an antioxidant.

8) Ellagic Acid is another acid with antioxidant properties, found in camu camu. It's been studied for anti-cancer effects, though the research is still very early. Some research also indicates that ellagic acid has anti-diabetic effects.

9) In one study, 20 male smokers drank camu camu juice or took vitamin C tablets daily for a week. The group who took camu camu showed a decrease in some markers for antioxidants and oxidative stress at the end of the study, compared to no change for those who had vitamin C tablets.

Camu camu berries are not exactly sold in your local North American supermarket, but you can include it in your diet in powder form. The powder can be used to flavor other foods like a smoothie or an ice-cream.

There are some concerns that camu camu can interfere with some chemotherapy medications. You should always let your doctor know about the supplements you are taking.

Maca

Maca is a root that originates in Peru. It's a tuber (like a potato) and offers an amazing energy boost for those with low energy. However, unlike coffee, maca offers energy in a non-caffeinated way that supports the body. Below, I've included an excerpt from a widely cited article written for *Natural News*, "Benefits of Maca Root: Find More Energy and Hormonal Balance" by Kim Evans:

Maca is a nutritionally dense super-food that contains high amounts of minerals, vitamins, enzymes, and all of the essential amino acids. Maca root is rich in B-vitamins, which are the energy vitamins, and maca is a vegetarian source of B-12. To boot, maca has high levels of bio-available calcium and magnesium and is great for remineralization.

Maca root helps balance our hormones and due to an over abundance of environmental estrogens, most people's hormones are a bit out of whack. Maca stimulates and nourishes the hypothalamus and pituitary glands which are the "master glands" of the body. These glands actually regulate the other glands, so when they are in balance, they can bring balance to the adrenal, thyroid, pancreas, ovarian, and testicular glands.

Instead of providing hormones to the body Maca works as an adaptogen, which means that it responds to different bodies' needs individually. If you're producing too much of a particular hormone, Maca will regulate the production downward. However, if you're producing too little, it'll regulate the production upward.

Hormones regulate many things including mood, growth, sexual development, and tissue function. Hormones also play a role in many diseases, like cancer and depression. Maca root has been shown to be beneficial for all sorts of hormonal problems including PMS, menopause, and hot flashes. Maca's also a fertility enhancer and is best known for improving libido and sexual function, especially in men. For this reason, it has earned the nickname "nature's Viagra."

Maca is a staple food in Peru and it doesn't have any toxic effects. However, occasionally some people DO experience adverse effects when they start taking maca. These symptoms may actually be due to detoxification. When a body is more accustomed to consuming processed and cooked foods, and suddenly starts taking in such a nutritionally dense supplement, the body will absorb the superior nutrients it needs and "throw off" the old junk it doesn't. If this happens, you might feel bad, but it generally lasts just a few days. You may also want to consider doing colon and liver cleansing before or while taking maca to quickly remove some of the waste your body is trying to eliminate.

Doing so will help with many of its adverse symptoms.

Shilajit

Shilajit, also known as silajit, salajeet or mumijo, momia and moomiyo or shargai, is a thick, sticky tar-like substance with a color ranging from white to dark brown (the latter is more common). It is sometimes found in Caucasus mountains, Altai Mountains, Tibet mountains, and the mountains of Gilgit Baltistan Pakistan. Shilajit is a blackish-brown exudation, of variable consistency, obtained from steep rocks of different formations found in the Himalayas. Shilajit is essentially microbially digested plant and mineral matter that has been incubated and pressurized for tens of thousands to millions of years through seismic and geological shifts.

As the Earth shifted, organic matter folded upon itself, trapping minerals between its layers. Eventually, the magnetized minerals made their way out through the crevices of the mountain in ionic and dual-ionic form. It is used in Ayurveda, the traditional Indian system of medicine. The composition of Shilajit has been investigated numerous times in both

India and the former USSR, and it depends on the location where it is found. It has been reported to contain at least 85 minerals in ionic form, as well as triterpenes, humic acid and fulvic acid. A similar substance from the Caucasus Mountains and the Altai Mountains is called *mumijo* (Russian).

Before we start talking about the benefits of Shilajit, I would like to point out that genuine Shilajit is RARE and VALUABLE. It is usually sold in powder form. There are countless companies trying to "sell" the consumer on countless benefits. However, the reality is very different. Behind many claims of benefits, there is nothing but marketing. The truth is that over 99% of products that are sold as shilajit are FAKE. Besides being counterfeit, they might just be—in the best-case scenario—soil extractions, or in the worst case scenario, a substance loaded with side effects from contaminants and for processing. Be careful when choosing the source.

Now about benefits. Caraka Saṃhit is the foundational body of knowledge of

Ayurveda. *Compendium of Caraka* is an ancient Indian medical text. It comprehensively addresses health, disease, and practice of medicine. Roughly 2,000 years old, it is still valid as a health maintenance manual. According to Caraka Samhita, there is no curable disease which can be treated without shilajit.

Modern-day science, when studying shilajit, has confirmed many ancient applications and demonstrated efficacy in vivo (living organisms) and in vitro (in the lab). The prominent names in Shilajit are the Soviet physician, A. Shakirov, and the Indian pharmaceutical chemist, S. Ghoshal. Much follow-up work was conducted by their followers, spanning countless physicians, biologists and chemists.

Shilajit is a compound with potent antioxidant properties. Below, I've included an overview of recent scientific findings as summarized by DetoxLab.org:

In an article called "Antilipid Peroxidative Property of Shilajit," researchers demonstrated that shilajit inhibits lipid peroxidation induced by cumene hydroperoxide and ADP/FE. It also reduced the rate of oxidation of reduced glutathione content and inhibited ongoing lipid peroxidation, induced by these agents immediately after its addition of the incubation system.

Processed extract of mumie efficiently traps hydroxyl radicals, NO and SO - radicals and can also regenerate ascorbic acid. Mumie is an inhibitor of lipid peroxidation induced by cumene hydroperoxide and ADP/Fe^{2+} complex in a dose-dependent manner. It decreases the rate of oxidation of reduced glutathione and inhibits ongoing lipid peroxidation, induced by these agents, immediately after its addition to the incubation system. Antiradical properties of mumie extract can be attributed to the presence of dibenzo-a-pyrones and fulvic acid. It is assumed that the therapeutic properties of some multicomponent preparations, containing mumijo in their composition, are caused by anti-radical properties of this humus matter. Mumie activates mitochondrial respiration but suppresses activity of succinate-oxidase and NADH-oxidase in mitochondrion (Igor Schepetkin 2002).

Genuine mumjo has a pronounced antimicrobial activity and on contact will neutralize different pathologic microbe strains such as staphylococci, streptococci, coliform bacteria, enterococci, and proteus. This was established by Dr. A. Shakirov in 1967-1969. Traditionally the substance was used to heal wounds producing pus (Igor Schepetkin 2002).

In a study called "Evaluation of the Anxiolytic Activity of NR-Anx-C" (a polyherbal formulation) in ethanol withdrawal-induced anxiety behavior in rats, a Shilajit-based formulation was used to control alcohol withdrawal symptoms in vivo. The study demonstrated that the use of the Shilajit-based herbal formulation is comparable in efficacy to the use of a pharmaceutical known as Alprazolam (also known as Xanax). The scientists managed to reduce anxiety in rats resulting from alcohol withdrawal symptoms (I. Mohan 2001).

It is rather exciting to me that it is naturally possible to support emotional health and stability with Shilajit. The frustrating part is that so far only Pürblack was capable of replicating such results naturally by claiming cumulative effects of alcohol neutralization and emotional resilience. Strange is the fact that if in the study one required several auxiliary herbs to create the effect of effective alcohol withdrawal, the leading

Shilajit brand on the market seems to manage replicate the effect simply using the Shilajit resin alone.

Mineral Pitch is a natural anabolic agent. It was traditionally used by Soviet sports and military to maintain health and increase strength and muscle mass while recuperating well and fast. The anabolic effect includes activation of an anabolic process on cellular and molecular levels in different organs and tissues. Researches have shown that a mumie extract accelerates the process of protein and nucleic acid synthesis, stimulates energy providing reactions in the liver, and promotes transport of minerals into muscle and bone tissue (Igor Schepetkin 2002).

Mumijo (A.k.a. Shilajit) is a nonspecific immune system stimulator. It proliferates lymphocytes and activates the macrophages. It was shown to accelerate regeneration of the immune system (lymphopoietic erythropoiesis). The resin restored the number of lymphocytes, peripheral blood, bone marrow and spleenmore rapidly (Igor Schepetkin 2002).

In "Effect of D-400, and Ayurvedic Herbal Formulation on Experimentally Induced Diabetes Mellitus," published in Phytotherapy Research volume 10 (1996). In this study, Shilajit was used as a part of an herbal formulation. Obviously the scientists knew that ancient physicians consistently used genuine Shilajit to treat diabetes often with herbs added to such formulations. In their study, they induced diabetes in vivo to animals and successfully demonstrated that upon application of Shilajit based formulation, diabetes can be successfully treated through repair and regeneration of endocrine pancreas. (S. K. Mitra 1996)

In a similar study called "Effect of Shilajit on blood glucose and lipid profile in alloxan-induced diabetic rats," scientists saw that Shilajit produced a significant reduction in blood glucose levels and also produced beneficial effects on the lipid profile. Even though in this study Shilajit was combined with pharmaceuticals in two doses out of three in each case results on blood sugar were beneficial (N. A. Trivedi 2004). The study confirmed the knowledge accumulated prior by Soviet physicians who did not use Shilajit (*Moomiyo* in Russian) as a self standing drug in medical therapy, but as a supplement to support efficacy of medical treatments. On the other hand, both studies also validated ancient therapies throughout Asian Shilajit/Moomiyo producing regions where the resin was used to actively control and treat people with diabetes prior to availability of modern-day pharmaceuticals.

Mumijo/Shilajit was traditionally used in Indian medicine to attenuate cerebral functional deficit, including amnesia, in geriatric patients. It was shown that Shilajit promoted learning and memory (Cho-Rok Jung 2002; Igor Schepetkin 2002).

In 2001 S. Ghosal with other two scientists published a paper called "Effects of Shilajit on the development of tolerance to morphine in mice." The scientists empirically demonstrated that administration of Shilajit on a daily basis inhibits development of tolerance to morphine induced analgesia. Morphine being an opioid is traditionally used to control pain. The downside of morphine use is the development of tolerance to it and constantly requiring higher doses leading to addiction to the compound. In the discussion part of the paper, one concluded that Shilajit could have a great potential as a prospective inhibitor of analgesic tolerance to morphine (P. Tiwari 2001).

Interestingly, most of the Shilajit on the market, except only one brand, does not demonstrate this effect. This is exactly why in order to get maximum benefits from your Mineral Pitch it is important to go for the brand that is not all hype, but demonstrates efficacy through unique quality. On the other hand, the problem with multiple brands and merchants offering "Shilajit" or imitations is that most of them will never show the efficacy of the substance originally tested in the lab environments.

"Glycine- and Gaba-mimetic Actions of Shilajit on the Substantia Gelatinosa Neurons of the Trigeminal Subnucleus Caudalis in Mice" was an in vitro study performed at the Department of Oral Physiology at Chonbuk National University, Korea. The research demonstrated that Shilajit mimics GABA and glycine receptors activation in the brain tissue. The research also suggested that it can be used to control certain types of pain (Hua Yin 2011). Moomie (Shilajit) may also contribute to stimulation of the human body to produce more of its own growth hormone and testosterone (Igor Schepetkin 2002).

Mumyo was traditionally used to detoxify and nourish. In a doctoral dissertation called "Moomiyo effect on tumor growth and creation of blood subjected to x-ray radiation," a Russian doctor Kaligin V. I. demonstrated the benefits of mineral pitch to counter negative effects of radiation sickness (Kaligin 1984). Unfortunately, this work is available only in Russian through the central scientific, medical library in Moscow. Antialergic Ghosal in 1888 and Bhattacharya in 1989 demonstrated significant anti-allergic activity of Shilajit stabilizing mast cells and decreasing degranulation (Igor Schepetkin 2002). Mineral Pitch (a.k.a. Moomiyo, Mumie, Shilajit, Shilajit) is a traditional anti-inflammatory agent. Greek physicians of antiquity used this medicine for various problems including arthritis and inflammation (Igor Schepetkin 2002).

The Mumie resin is an excellent tool against inflammation. Indeed, traditionally, it was used in folk medicine to treat people with inflammatory issues. Multiple modern scientific studies demonstrated its efficacy. As an auxiliary, it was conventionally used to support patients with paradentosis, osteoarthritis, rheumatoid arthritis, ankylosing spondylitis, and cervical spondylosis. Soviet doctors have routinely used it to clean wounds from necrotic tissues, granulation, epithelization, and decrease the period of wound healing. In the lab, Shilajit has demonstrated to be a powerful tool to suppress artificially induced inflammation (Igor Schepetkin 2002).

"Complement-fixing Activity of Fulvic Acid from Shilajit and Other Natural Sources" was published by an international group of scientists from the Montana State University who demonstrated that Shilajit is a highly potent complement fixing agent. Even though the study was performed in vitro, in a way it revealed why Shilajit was traditionally used in folk medicine for the treatment of a variety of disorders, including syndromes involving excessive complement activation. The study established that multiple fractions of Shilajit are products of broken down polysaccharides, and suggested that such extracts from different plans would enhance wound healing and have a potential to treat inflammatory disease (Igor A. Schepetkin 2009).

Moomiyo activates mitochondrial respiration but suppresses activity of succinate: oxidase and NADH-oxidase in mitochondrion. It induces an increase in superoxide dismutase, catalase, and glutathione peroxidase activities in adults as well. This means that while increasing production of energy through a cellular respiration, the substance simultaneously protects from damage that usually goes along with increased production of energy (Igor Schepetkin 2002).

In the article "Medical Drugs From Humus Matter: Focus on Moomijo," researchers I. Schepetkin, A. Khlebnikov and Byoung Se Kwon discuss medicinal properties of Moomiyo (also known as Mumie, Shilajit, Salajeet, etc.). According to the article the substance was traditionally used in Asian herbal medicine both inwardly and outwardly against injuries, bone fractures, dislocations, diseases of skin, diseases of peripheral nervous system, and also as a soothing and anti-inflammatory agent (Igor Schepetkin 2002). In the same article, it is noted that the resin will regenerate damaged bones approximately 2 times faster than they normally would. This effect was used by Soviet surgeons consistently for many years (Igor Schepetkin 2002). Moomie showed to be highly effective in the treatment of thermal burns and stimulation of hepatic regeneration (Igor Schepetkin 2002).

Mineral Pitch Resin (Shilajit, Moomiyo, Salajeet, etc.) is a known enhancing cognition. It can protect the neuron tissue in vitro (Anna Aiello 2008) . As the physical performance enhancer, it has been used to promote better strength, recovery, and muscular hypertrophy. (Bucci 2000)

To summarize, the latest research confirmed benefits of shilajit as it being anti-allergic, anti-diabetic, anti-fungal, anti-inflammatory for arthritis and rheumatism, anti-oxidant, anti-viral, Alzheimer's prevention, cognitive and memory enhancer, fertility increases, motility and count, high altitude problems/hypoxia, sickness, lethargy, depression, influenza/common cold, mental and physical rejuvenation or anti aging benefits, pain relief and injury repair, stress and anxiety reduction, and ulcer repair.

Shilajit could be one of the great superfood wonders that not many people have heard about.

Royal Jelly

Although royal jelly does come from bees, it should not be confused with bee pollen or bee venom: royal jelly is entirely different. So what is it? As described by WindowBee.com:

Royal jelly is a milky secretion produced by worker honeybees. It typically contains about 60% to 70% water, 12% to 15% proteins, 10% to 16% sugar, 3% to 6% fats, and 2% to 3% vitamins, salts, and amino acids. Its composition varies depending on geography and climate. This product gets its name from the fact that bees use it for the development and nurturing of the queen bees.

Royal jelly is used for asthma, hay fever, liver diseases, pancreatitis, sleep troubles (insomnia), premenstrual syndrome (PMS), stomach ulcers, kidney disease, bone fractures, menopausal symptoms, skin disorders, and high cholesterol. It is also used as a general health tonic, for fighting the effects of aging, and for boosting the immune system. Some people apply royal jelly directly to the skin as a tonic or to the scalp to encourage hair growth. In animals, royal jelly seems to have some activity against tumors and the development of "hardening of the arteries."

Here are the health benefits of royal jelly that are supported by science:

1) When your cells oxidize, YOU oxidize. That leads to greater instances of cancer, heart disease, and other degenerative conditions. We've all seen a peeled apple turn brown within minutes—and that is literally what happens to your cells over your lifetime. Scientists have discovered that certain foods have massive amounts of antioxidants that can slow and can even stop this process. Royal jelly is one of these foods. As reported in the *Journal of Agricultural Food Chemistry* in

2008, royal jelly contains high amounts of several antioxidants, especially when it is fresh and raw.

2) Because royal jelly has been indicated to have immuno-modulatory potential for humans, a group of scientists at the University of the Ryukyus in Japan undertook a study to determine whether it could alter the development of systemic autoimmunity in mice.

Autoimmunity is a state in which the body's immune system attacks itself. Diseases like rheumatoid arthritis and many other allergies are autoimmune disorders. These mice were genetically predisposed to get lupus, a serious autoimmune disorder. During the study, the scientists found that the mice that were getting the royal jelly supplement saw a significant delay in getting lupus and once they did get it, they lived significantly longer than the mice that didn't get the supplement. While humans aren't mice, this study certainly supports the many testimonials of people who have reported using royal jelly to boost or balance their immune systems.

3) A lot of people often report that they experience a mild euphoria or feeling of clarity upon taking high quality, fresh royal jelly. A study from Gifu Pharmaceutical University in Japan has shed some light on why this happens. Scientists fed a toxic compound to rats that was designed to kill brain cells and then gave them royal jelly. They found that not only did the royal jelly protect the brain, but it also stimulated cognitive function and repair to the brain.

4) Royal jelly also has liver protective abilities. I've met many people with toxic or impaired livers and it is a very challenging health situation, which can often lead to liver cancer. Simply drinking tap water today will expose your liver to over 200 toxic compounds alone. This makes the protective effects of royal jelly even more important. Scientists at the University of Erciyes in Turkey fed royal jelly to mice that had been given a liver toxin. They found that the administration of royal jelly as a

liver protective agent for only seven days exhibited a marked protective effect on liver tissue from the toxin.

5) A tremendous amount of research is now showing that chronic inflammation is one of the root causes of heart disease and other degenerative diseases such as Alzheimers disease, arthritis, and even some cancers. A group of scientists at the Hayashibara Biochemical Laboratories in Japan decided to test the anti-inflammatory activity of royal jelly. They tested for pro-inflammatory cytokines such as TNF-alpha, IL-6, and IL-1. High levels of these compounds indicate high levels of inflammation. The scientists found that the administration of royal jelly suppressed these pro-inflammatory compounds and concluded that RJ has anti-inflammatory actions. So, if you have a history of heart disease or Alzheimer's disease in your family—or better yet, you've had your IL-6 levels tested by your doctor and they are elevated, royal jelly is likely an excellent supplement for you.

6) Scientists at the Department of Pharmacology at Nihon University in Japan set out to discover whether royal jelly can augment wound healing. They fed rats various amounts of the Royal jelly daily and found that it showed anti-inflammatory activity by decreasing exudation and collagen formation. The jelly also shortened the healing period of skin lesions, enough to convince the scientists that royal jelly is able to augment wound healing. This comes as no surprise to those of us who have used royal jelly for skin health over the years.

7) It contains specific nutrients and vitamins that support skin renewal such as flavonoids, nucleic acid, decanoic acid, enzymes, and hormones. It also contains numerous vitamins and minerals such as vitamins B1, B2, B3, B5, B6, acetyl-choline and zinc, all of which are excellent for the skin. Studies indicate that the acids found in royal jelly contribute to its collagen production and promotion.

8) Earlier studies have shown that royal jelly works like insulin. However, so far there had been no clinical trials to support these findings. A group of German doctors at the Justus-Liebig University Hospital in Germany had 20 volunteers undergo the standardized oral glucose tolerance test (OGTT) and afterwards, a second OGTT after ingestion of 20g of Royal jelly. The doctors found that after two hours, the serum sugar levels of the 20 volunteers were much lower after taking the 20g of Royal jelly than when they didn't take it. So, if you have any type of blood sugar issue, try supplementing with royal jelly (if you are on insulin or Glucagon, make sure you monitor your levels carefully, as royal jelly will reduce your sugar level).

9) A group of Japanese scientists hypothesized that royal jelly may have beneficial effects on osteoporosis. After conducting a study on rats and in a test tube, the doctors found that RJ may prevent osteoporosis by enhancing intestinal calcium absorption. This makes it an effective

preventative aid for osteoporosis. It makes a lot of sense to supplement with royal jelly along with your calcium and vitamin D if you are suffering from osteoporosis or have a history of it in your family. According to this study, it will enhance your body's ability to absorb the calcium and in turn deposit it within your bone structure.

10) A group of scientists at the Kyushu University in Japan looked at the protective effect of royal jelly on breast cancer cells. In the study, the scientists found an anti-environmental estrogen effect of royal jelly. Bisphenol A (BPA) is an environmental estrogen found in many plastics that stimulates the proliferation of human breast cancer MCF-7 cells. The study found that royal jelly inhibited the growth promoting effect of BPA on breast cancer MCF-7 cells, even though it did not affect the proliferation of cells in the absence of BPA. We are all exposed to dozens of cancer causing environmental estrogens every day through our drinking water, our cosmetics, plastics, and our food. You would be

wise to protect yourself from these cancers with a daily dose of fresh royal jelly.

11) A group of researchers in Japan decided to examine the effects of royal jelly on blood cholesterol levels in 15 volunteers. They gave half the volunteers six grams of royal jelly per day for four weeks. Those taking the RJ saw their total cholesterol and low-density lipoprotein (LDL) decreased significantly compared with those who didn't get the royal jelly. HDL (the good cholesterol) levels didn't change in either group, nor did triglyceride levels. So, it appears that royal jelly lowers bad cholesterol and total cholesterol while not harming good cholesterol levels.

I think it's also important to keep in mind where this RJ comes from. If it's from GMO-laden fields with toxic flowers, the bees will create a concentration of those GMO chemicals...and that could be harmful for your health. But, if it's organic or wild raw non-toxic RJ, then it could be beneficial. Keep in mind that all superfoods and supplements that I mentioned here are awesome—but it doesn't mean that you should go and buy and use all of them at once.

Just pick one or two that work for you, and remember: less is more. This means that if you eat the optimal health diet, you don't really need any supplements or super foods at all. Any and all super food should be looked at as only a temporary crutch. Your body can totally detox and re-balance itself and do an excellent job on its own, provided that you don't put any other extra toxins in the system and stay out of its way when it is healing. Everyone is different and has different needs and requirements depending on which toxins they hold and how toxic they are.

Chlorella

Chlorella is a single-celled fresh-water algae and one of the most heavily researched algae across the globe. Some even call it a "near-perfect" food, as research through the years have identified an astounding range of health benefits. While well-known for its ability to detoxify your body by binding to toxins and carrying them out of your system, chlorella can be used for much, more more. It works great in detoxifying your body from heavy metals. I prefer buying chlorella in a form of a pill (make sure it's only organic and pure broken wall cell chlorella and has no additives).

Here's a sampling of some of the health benefits associated with this green algae:

- Repairing nerve tissues
- Increasing your energy levels
- Enhancing your immune system
- Normalizing your blood sugar
- Improving digestion
- Normalizing your blood pressure

- Promoting healthy pH levels in your gut, which helps good bacteria to thrive
- Removing potentially toxic metals from your body
- Enhancing your ability to focus and concentrate
- Eliminating bad breath

Chlorella can also be of benefit to vegetarians and vegans looking for proteins and B vitamins from a non-animal source. About 60 percent of it is protein. Because it contains all the essential amino acids your body needs, it is called a "complete protein." Chlorella is also rich in GABA, folate, vitamin B12, and iron.

Below, I've incoporated some research from the Society of Natural Therapists and Researchers to discuss some health conditions chlorella may help prevent or treat:

1) **Insulin resistance**—Researchers discovered that chlorella has the ability to improve fructose-induced insulin sensitivity. Excessive fructose consumption is the number

one cause of insulin resistance and type 2 diabetes. In a study, a group of rats were given chlorella three times a day for five days, after being fed fructose-rich chow for four weeks. Chlorella brought their elevated glucose-insulin values back to normal. The authors concluded that, "Oral administration of chlorella has the ability to improve insulin sensitivity, which may be used as an adjuvant therapy for patients with insulin resistance."

2) **Detoxification**—This is particularly helpful when used in conjunction with an infrared sauna and taken two hours before you go in the sauna. This way, the chlorella will be in your intestine and ready to bind to the toxins that are released when you are in the sauna. It will bind irreversibly to the toxins, and will be safely excreted when you have bowel movement. But it works like magic whether you have time to go to the sauna or not. If you take it on a daily basis, it will help you detox faster and more efficiently. It is particularly crucial for systemic mercury elimination, because the majority of mercury is rid through your stool.

Once the burden of mercury is lowered from your intestines, mercury from other body tissues will more readily migrate into your intestines where chlorella will work to remove it. You can also add cilantro, which works as a synergetic detoxification aid along with the chlorella. This combination is particularly useful to take when you're consuming seafood, as most are invariably contaminated with heavy metals and chemicals. Ideally, you would take it with the meal so that the chlorella can bind directly to the toxins while they are in your gut, before they are absorbed into your body. In order to optimize heavy metal detox, you will want to take minimum four grams of chlorella every day, for at least the whole year.

3) **Diabetes**—Additional evidence supporting the theory that chlorella can improve insulin sensitivity can be found in an earlier study. The algae were found to improve insulin sensitivity and glucose uptake in the liver in type 1 diabetic rats. The authors suggest that chlorella's hypoglycemic effects may be due to improved glucose uptake in the liver and

the soleus muscles. Another mechanism may be related to decreased levels of nonesterified fatty acids (NEFA), since insulin sensitivity is usually blunted by elevated NEFA in type 1 diabetes.

4) **Hypertension**—The results from a placebo-controlled, double-blind published study suggest that chlorella can significantly decrease high-normal blood pressure and borderline hypertension. The authors proposed that it might be a beneficial dietary supplement for preventing hypertension, with no apparent adverse side effects.

5) **Anemia, proteinuria, and edema in pregnancy**—Pregnancy-induced hypertension and anemia are common, and potentially dangerous. One of the primary causes for these conditions is the woman's nutritional status. It was found in a published study that chlorella may help improve both of these conditions in pregnant women, likely due to its high folate, B12 and iron content. Subjects took six grams of chlorella per day, starting somewhere between the 12th

to the 18th week of gestation, until delivery. The chlorella group had significantly lower rates of anemia, compared to the control group. They also had fewer incidences of proteinuria and edema, which are two symptoms associated with pregnancy-induced hypertension. The authors concluded that, "Chlorella supplement may be useful as a resource of natural folate, vitamin B-12 and iron for pregnant women."

6)   **Fibromyalgia**—Although the individual results were varied, it may be worth considering chlorella if you suffer with fibromyalgia to decrease pain intensity.

7) **Liver cancer**—A study published in 2009 discovered that chlorella triggers cell death (apoptosis) in rat liver cancer cells, which suggests it may be useful in the prevention of liver cancer. The authors concluded that, "Our study shows that chlorella has a definite chemopreventive effect by inducing apoptosis via decreasing the expression of Bcl-2 and increasing the

expression of caspase 8 in hepatocarcinogenesis-induced rats."

Some side effects may occur. As your body begins detoxing, you may start to experience slight nausea, and/or mild diarrhea. Should these symptoms become irritating, you can lower your dose and slowly build back up. As the toxins slowly leave your system, the side effects should fade away as well.

Chlorella's detoxing properties come from its cellular membrane, but the cellular wall is indigestible in our stomachs. This is why you will see many chlorella products state that they contain a "broken cell wall," which means that the chlorella has been broken down to a digestible form. Don't waste your money buying a chlorella product that does not have a broken cell wall, as you will not be able to reap any of the benefits.

Whether you want to help reduce your toxic burden, prevent a particular health ailment, or just boost overall nutrition, I believe chlorella can be a phenomenal addition to a healthy diet. Chlorella takes away bad smells and even morning breath once you work your way up to a higher dose. You will be surprised that when you start taking higher doses on a daily basis, you won't even have morning breath anymore, and your excrement won't have a bad odor.

But be very careful with it, as it is a very strong detoxifier. Chlorella might make you sick if you are very toxic and have a lot of heavy metals stored in your body tissues.

Yacon Syrup

Yacon syrup is extracted from the roots of the Yacon plant. The Yacon plant, also called *Smallanthus sonchifolius*, grows natively in the Andes Mountains in South America. This plant has been eaten and used for medicinal purposes for hundreds of years in South America. Local people believed it to have powerful medicinal properties, resulting in improvements in diabetes and helping with kidney and digestive disorders.

The Yacon root looks kind of similar to a sweet potato. The juices from the roots are extracted, then filtered and evaporated in a chemical-free manufacturing process that resembles the way Maple syrup is made. The final product is a sweet-tasting syrup, with a dark color and a consistency similar to molasses. I am not sure that it would be considered as a raw food, but it does have a beneficial effect on the human system, and is a much better choice than refined sugar.

The active ingredient in Yacon Syrup is fructooligosaccharides (FOS). Yacon syrup is one of the best dietary sources of fructooligosaccharides. The exact amount may vary between batches, but Yacon syrup usually contains roughly about 40-50% fructooligosaccharides. These are sugar molecules that are connected in a way that makes them unrecognizable by the digestive system. Even though these sugars can stimulate the taste buds, humans can not digest them. Yacon syrup does contain a small amount of digestible sugars, including fructose, glucose and sucrose. The rest of it is fructooligosaccharides and a fiber called inulin. Because a large part of Yacon syrup isn't digested, it has only a third of the caloric value of sugar, about 133 calories per 100 grams, or 20 calories per tablespoon. For this reason, it can be used as a low-calorie alternative to sugar.

The fructooligosaccharides eventually reach the large intestine, where they feed the friendly bacteria in the digestive system. This is where Yacon syrup works its magic... in the gut. The friendly bacteria in the gut are actually incredibly important for the health of our bodies. Having the "right" types is associated with a lower risk of diabetes, better immunity, and improved brain function to name a few. When the bacteria digest the fructooligosaccharides, they also produce short-chain fatty acids that have powerful anti-obesity effects, at least in rats. There is also some evidence that fructooligosaccharides can lower the hunger hormone ghrelin, helping to reduce appetite. Keep in mind that Yacon is not the only food that contains fructooligosaccharides. They are also found in smaller amounts in artichokes, onions, garlic, leeks, and various other plant foods.

When it comes to weight loss, pretty much all of the claims behind Yacon syrup rest on just one study called "Yacon syrup: Beneficial effects on obesity and insulin resistance in humans." This study was a double-blind, placebo-controlled clinical trial. The study included participants that were 55 obese women with cholesterol problems and a history of constipation. The women were split into two groups: 40 women took Yacon syrup, while 15 women took another type of syrup with no active ingredients (placebo). All of them were advised to eat a low-fat diet and to mildly restrict their calories. The study went on for 120 days, about four months. The results showed that after a study period of 120 days, the women in the Yacon syrup group had lost 33 pounds (15 kg) on average. At the same time, the placebo group gained an average of 3.5 pounds (1.6 kg). They also saw reductions in waist circumference. The women in the Yacon syrup group lost 3.9 inches, or 10 centimeters, off of their waist, while there was no significant change in the placebo group. There were several other effects also noted in the Yacon syrup group:

- Their Body Mass Index (BMI) went from obese to overweight (34 to 28).
- Their stool frequency increased from 0.28 per day to 0.99 per day, effectively curing them of constipation.

- Fasting insulin levels went down by 42%.

- Insulin resistance, a major risk factor for diabetes and heart disease, decreased by 67%.

- LDL (the "bad") cholesterol went from 137 mg/dL to 97.5 mg/dL (a 29% decrease).

Overall, the women taking the Yacon syrup had dramatic improvements in both body weight and metabolic health, while the women taking the placebo stayed pretty much the same. Studies on other types of soluble fiber have shown some amount of weight loss, but not nearly this impressive.

Due to the high amount of fructooligosaccharides, Yacon syrup has various other health benefits, including reduced symptoms of constipation— a very common health problem. In one study, Yacon syrup reduced the transit time through the digestive tract from 60 to 40 hours and increased stool frequency from 1.1 to 1.3 per day. There is also some evidence that it can lower blood sugar, although this needs to be studied a lot more. Fructooligosaccharides effectively function as soluble, fermentable fibers, which have various other benefits. Yacon syrup is also high in antioxidants and potassium.

There are still some side effects to consider when it comes to eating Yacon syrup, esepecially if you have too much in one sitting. These side effects are like what you might experience if you consume more fiber than you usually would. Once a large quantity of Yacon syrup is in the intestine, it can create gaseous reactions, causing nausea, diarrhea, flatulence, and general discomfort in your digestive tract. As a result, your best bet is to start taking small doses of Yacon syrup before breakfast, lunch, and dinner. Start with one teaspoon and work your way up to two.

Yacon syrup can also be used as a natural sweetener, but it's not suitable for cooking or baking. Temperatures above 248°F will cause the fructooligosaccharides to break down. And make sure that you are only using Yacon syrup that has no additives and is 100% pure.

Because Yacon syrup is high in fructooligosaccharides (FOS) and low in glucemic number, it is great to use it if you need to rebalance your gut flora, if you have a problem with Candida, or if you have other intestinal flora issues.

Flax seed oil

The first time I heard about flax seed oil was when I was researching about what could be done to help my allergies without using any chemicals and pills, and I came across flax seed oil. It seemed to me that it helps to alleviate the symptoms of allergies. I decided to try it, and it really helped me with my allergies. I wouldn't say that it cured me, but it definitely did help. In short, any allergy is a high toxicity buildup in your body that makes your system to overreact to things that are not a threat, because the body sees them as a threat. Flax seed oil helps to de-congest the intestines and that might be one of the reasons why symptoms of allergies get better (toxins get to exit the body instead of sitting stagnant in your intestines). See the synopis below from HerbWisdom.com for more details on flax seed and its healing properties:

A rich source of healing compounds, flaxseed (also called linseed) has been cultivated for more than 7000 years. First cultivated in Europe, the plant's brown seeds were regularly used to prepare balms for inflamed skin and healing slurries for constipation. Rich in essential fatty acids, or EFAs, flaxseed oil is used to prevent and treat heart disease, to relieve a variety of inflammatory disorders and hormone-related problems, and many more problems including infertility.

A source of fiber for linen fabric since ancient times, the slender flax plant also boasts a long history as a healing herb. Today, flaxseeds are best known for the therapeutic oil that is derived by pressing them. Flaxseed oil has earned a solid reputation for treating a range of ailments ranging from heart disease to lupus.

The essential fatty acids (Omega oils) in flaxseed oil are one of its key healing components. Essential Fatty Acids (EFAs) are particularly valuable because the body needs them to function properly, but cannot manufacture them on its own [so they say]. Essential fatty acids work throughout the body to protect cell membranes, keeping them efficient at admitting healthy substances while barring damaging ones.

One of the EFAs in flaxseed oil, alpha-linolenic acid, is known as an omega-3 fatty acid. Like the omega-3s found in fish, it appears to reduce the risk of heart disease and numerous other ailments. Flaxseed oil is an excellent source of omega-3s: just 1 teaspoon contains about 2.5 grams, equivalent to more than twice the amount most people get through their diets. Flaxseeds also contain omega-6 fatty acids in the form of linoleic acid. Omega-6s are the same healthy fats found in vegetable oils.

Flaxseed oil only contains these alpha-linolenic acid (Omega 3 oils), and not the fiber or lignan components that the whole plant contains. Therefore, flaxseed oil provides the Omega 3 benefits, such as lipid-lowering properties, but not the laxative or anti-cancer properties. In my personal experience, it seems that flaxseed oil regulates the bowel movement, but it is not laxative.It makes you go to the bathroom if you are congested, but does not cause diarrhea.

Whole flaxseeds (not the extracted oil) are a rich source of lignans (phytoestrogens), substances that appear to positively affect hormone-related problems. Lignans may also be useful in preventing certain cancers and combating specific bacteria, fungi, and viruses, including those that cause cold sores and shingles.

According to the same article, some of the wide-ranging benefits of flax seeds are stated below.

- **Lowering cholesterol, protects against heart disease and control high blood pressure:** Several studies indicate that flaxseed oil, as well as ground flaxseeds, can lower cholesterol, thereby significantly reducing the risk of heart disease. Taking flaxseed oil may also protect against angina (chest pain) and high blood pressure. In addition, a five-year study done recently at Boston's Simmons College found that flaxseed oil might be useful in preventing a second heart attack. It may also help prevent elevated blood pressure by inhibiting inflammatory reactions that cause artery-hardening plaque and poor circulation.

- **Countering inflammation associated with gout, lupus and fibrocystic breasts:** Omega-3 fatty acids appear to limit the inflammatory reaction associated with these conditions. In cases of lupus, flaxseed oil not only reduces inflammation in the joints, skin and kidneys, but also lowers cholesterol levels that may be elevated by the disease. Taking flaxseed oil for gout may lessen the often sudden and severe joint pain or swelling that is a symptom of this condition. In addition, the ability of omega-3 fatty acids to boost the absorption of iodine (a mineral often found in low levels in women suffering from fibrocystic breasts) makes flaxseed oil potentially valuable for treating this often painful condition.

- **Controling constipation, hemorrhoids, diverticular disorders and gallstones:** As they are high in dietary fiber, ground flaxseeds can help ease the passage of stools and thus relieve constipation, hemorrhoids, and diverticular disease. In those with diverticular disease, flaxseeds may also keep intestinal pouches free of waste and thus keep potential infection at bay. Taken for inflammatory bowel disease, flaxseed oil can help to calm inflammation and repair any intestinal tract damage. In addition, the oil may prevent painful gallstones from developing and even dissolve existing stones.

- **Treating acne, eczema, psoriasis, sunburn and rosacea:** The essential fatty acids in flaxseed oil are largely responsible for its skin-healing powers. Red, itchy patches of eczema, psoriasis and rosacea often respond to the EFA's anti-inflammatory actions and overall skin-soothing properties. Sunburned skin may heal faster when treated with the oil as well. In cases of acne, the EFAs encourage thinning of the oily sebum that clogs pores.

- **Promoting healthy hair and nails:** The abundant omega-3 fatty acids in flaxseed oil have been shown to contribute to healthy hair growth (in fact, low levels of these acids may cause dry and lackluster locks). Hair problems exacerbated by psoriasis or eczema of the scalp may respond to the skin-revitalizing and anti-inflammatory actions of flaxseed oil as well. Similarly, the oil's EFAs work to nourish dry or brittle nails, stopping them from cracking or splitting.

- **Minimizing nerve damage that causes numbness and tingling as well as other disorders:** The EFAs in flaxseed oil assist in the transmission of nerve impulses, making the oil potentially valuable in treating conditions of numbness and tingling. The oil's nerve-nourishing actions may also help in the treatment of Parkinson's disease — a degenerative disorder of the nervous system —and protect against the nerve damage associated with diabetes and multiple sclerosis.

- **Reducing risk of cancer and guard against the effects of aging:** The lignans in flaxseed appear to play a role in protecting against breast, colon, prostate, and perhaps even skin cancer. Although further studies are needed, research undertaken at the University of Toronto indicates that women with breast cancer, regardless of the degree of cancer invasiveness, may benefit from treatment with flaxseed. Interestingly, the lignans may protect against various effects of ageing as well.

- **Treating menopausal symptoms, menstrual cramps, female infertility and endometriosis:** Because the hormone-balancing lignans and plant estrogens (phytoestrogens) in flaxseed help stabilize a woman's estrogen-progesterone ratio, they can

487

have beneficial effects on the menstrual cycle, and relieve the hot flashes of perimenopause and menopause. Flaxseed may also improve uterine function and thus treat fertility problems. In addition, the essential fatty acids in flaxseed have been shown to block production of prostaglandins, a hormone-like substances that when released in excess amounts during menstruation, can cause heavy bleeding associated with endometriosis.

- **Fighting prostate problems, male infertility and impotence:** The EFAs in flaxseed oil may help to prevent swelling and inflammation of the prostate, the small gland located below the bladder in males that tends to enlarge with age. Symptoms of such enlargement, such as urgency to urinate, may lessen as a result. The EFAs also play a role in keeping sperm healthy, which may be of value in treating male infertility. In addition to that, they can improve blood flow to the penis, a boon for those suffering from impotence.

In general, I noticed a very positive effect on me after taking one tablespoon of flax seed oil with dinner when I started my transition to raw vegan foods. I was taking it for about eight months before I decided that I had enough. When your body craves it, you will automatically want to take it. It has a very tasty, nutty flavor to it. It works great on green salads as a dressing. But once your body is done with it, the cravings stop. That's a good time to listen to your body and know that you need to take a break. You will never go wrong by listening to your body's natural signals! Also, keep in mind that it has to be refrigerated at all times. When you buy it at the store, make sure that it is in the refrigerated section.

MSM (Methyl Sulfonyl Methane)

This is a pure and beneficial form of organic sulphur, a naturally occurring nutrient found in every living organism. It is not related to common sulphurs, sulphates or sulphites (which are irritants), and is not yellow as people always think of sulphur. In its purest form, it is white crystals and is a naturally occurring mineral. MSM is found in the oceans, rain water, in all living things, and in amino acids such as, methionine, taurine, cysteine, and cystine. In his book *Eating for Beauty*, David Wolfe discusses the beautifying effects of MSM in detail. He also mentions that MSM is great for detoxifying from mercury.

MSM is a beneficial dietary supplement of sulphur. Its toxicity rating is the same as water. It has the lowest levels of toxicity in biology. It can safely be taken with other medications, although it is always recommended that a doctor be consulted before you take anything in addition to your prescription medication.

It is best to start with the lowest dose and then slowly build up. The lowest recommended beneficial amount is of 1,500mg per day, in two or three doses, although people were taking as much as 10,000mg quite safely in the specific treatment of arthritis (although it also benefits skin, hair, and nails). Scientific tests were also done where doses of 8g per kilogram of body weight have been used with no after effects. This goes on to prove how safe this product is. Particular benefit is to be had if a high dose of vitamin C (2000mg) is also taken.

I recommend to take MSM starting from ¼ of a teaspoon and slowly increasing the dose all the way up to a tablespoon (please seek advice with your doctor before starting taking anything new). The reason for this is that MSM has quite the detoxifying effect. It can also be fairly stimulating. In some cases, it may produce palpitations while some people also experience anxiety attacks. I recommend that you start as low as possible in order to benefit from it without side effects, and choose as good a brand as you can. It needs to be a very pure form. Please watch out for anti-caking agents like silicone dioxide that are added to the powder (it is not good to eat sand or other toxic agents with MSM).

Detoxing effects of MSM may produce gastrointestinal cramping, or an upset stomach, or headaches and diarrhea. I personally haven't experienced any of the above mentioned symptoms—in fact, I didn't actually feel anything while I was taking it. You may also get a Herxheimer reaction and strong detox effects, so drinking plenty of water in order to help flush this through is recommended. This is not the case for everyone, but in the cases of those with chronic health problems or underlying unresolved issues, old viruses/pathogens may come to the surface as with any strong detox as the die off from these is sent into the bloodstream. Those with any sort of liver dysfunction may struggle a bit, as a sluggish liver does not remove toxins as efficiently as a fully functional liver.

MSM is a beneficial supplement for cleansing, detoxing, pain management, chronic illness, skin, hair, and nails—but like any supplement, you need to go very slowly. It can take as long as two months to see a result (or as little as a week), but this is the case with all supplements and is probably the reason people give up. Please remember that you need to take any supplement for at least two to four months before you will feel its benefits, as the body needs to absorb and use the nutrient over a period of time.

MSM is the vital component in the formation of keratin, collagen and elastin, giving flexibility, tone and strength to our muscles, bones, joints, internal membranes, skin, hair and nails. It is also a free radical scavenger. MSM can also give a relief from swelling and inflammation. Research on arthritis pain symptoms has shown that symptoms improve when taking MSM. It can also be beneficial as part of a care plan for fibromyalgia.

Our skin, hair, and nails all contain sulphur and it is this that you smell if you have ever burnt your hair. MSM has a beautifying effect on hair, skin, and nails, as it smoothes the skin because of its collagen-building effects, strengthens hair and nails, and causes accelerated growth. It is an essential component of all connective tissue. David Wolfe states in his book *Eating for Beauty* that sulphur is the most beautifying of all nutrients and is the best cosmetic in the world! Sulphur can clear acne sometimes in a matter of weeks. Its effects are accelerated by adding vitamin C. The best form of vitamin C would be found in Camu Camu, or Acerola cherry.

Due to processed food and modern farming techniques, scientists believe that we have become deficient in this very important mineral and that the amount now in our diet is negligible. Therefore, it is recommended that a daily supplement is taken. There have been no observed side effects in patients taking this supplement over a 20-year time span.

MSM benefits all of us, but especially those suffering from arthritis and joint problems and inflammation. It also helps migraine sufferers and athletes in reducing or eliminating muscle cramps. It is good for fibromyalgia and other chronic illnesses as part of nutritional therapy. It is also beneficial in reducing wrinkles and promoting strong hair, skin and nails—and for this reason alone, is recommended for women from an anti-aging aspect. It supports the immune system, so it is beneficial for those needing immune support and for allergy sufferers suffering from respiratory congestion, inflammation and discharge of mucus. It also assists the liver in producing additional choline, helps increase the body's ability to produce insulin, boosts the metabolism of carbohydrates, and supports general well-being, including mental alertness and wound healing.

Sulfur regulates the balance of sodium and potassium in our cells. It relieves pain and inflammation, and is detoxifying. It also helps stabilize blood sugar and reduces lactic acid build up reducing cramps. It alleviates allergies, and is excellent for healing of chronic gum problems as an ongoing treatment when taken with vitamin C. MSM is also available as a lotion for tropical application at Raw Gaia, as well as MSM Beauty Spray, which has amazing skin reconstructive abilities. It is best to take the powder, starting with a low dose of a teaspoon and building up to around two to three tablespoons a day (or to tolerance). It is best consumed in water, so dissolve the powder in a glass of water—although I should warn you that it doesn't taste good.

Sulphur is rich in many foods, but cooking will destroy it. It can be found in garlic, onion, mustard, horseradish, broccoli, cabbage, brussels sprouts, radishes, watercress, spirulina, maca, pumpkin seeds, kale, rocket, hemp seeds, and chilli peppers. Eating an abundance of these foods in their raw state is also beneficial for their sulphur residues. Keep in mind that overeating will cause gas in the intestine, so combine it with oils to "soften" the effect. You can also combine sulfur-rich foods with salty vegetables like spinach, celery, or chard.

All in all, MSM is a beneficial supplement. The powder form is best, although tablets and capsules are also available. It is best consumed in the morning and early afternoon, as taking in the evening can produce unwanted energizing effects before bedtime.

Natural Cellular Defense –

Liquid Zeolite

Zeolites are naturally occurring crystalline minerals commonly found in rock deposits. These micro-porous compounds are formed by the crystallization of volcanic rock and ash when they come in contact with salt water over millions of years. Zeolite selectively attracts and binds toxic particles (in the forms of heavy metals, radioactive particles, some small viral particles, volatile organic compounds and many other chemicals) within or onto itself. These toxic particles may be contributing factors to chronic illness or fatigue. Zeolites safely removes them and their negative impacts on overall health and wellness. It is a great way for removing mercury out of your system.

The molecular structure of zeolites actually resembles a honeycomb. The cell carries an overall negative charge and, like a magnet, attracts positively charged particles.

When prepared as a supplement, zeolites can be "pre-loaded" with beneficial electrolyte nutrients such as calcium, sodium, magnesium, potassium, and iron. When positively charged ions outside the zeolite structure (such as heavy metals, free radicals, and viral sub particles) come into contact with zeolites, they simply exchange places with one of the less-tightly bound "pre-loaded" nutrients that are already there. This exchange of particles is what gives the compound its unique detoxifying properties.

I'd like to mention some benefits of using zeolites:

1) Supports Liver and Kidney Health – The liver and kidneys are the body's two primary detoxification organs. They are responsible for filtering out the "bad stuff." Zeolites can help lessen the burden of detoxification on these organs, thereby supporting their healthy function.

2) Improves Digestive Function –
Scientists have found that zeolites may help to
relieve diarrhea and possibly enhance the
absorption of nutrients in the digestive tract.
Zeolites may also aid in normalizing bowel
movements, acid reflux, leaky gut, and other
intestinal disorders.

3) Relieves from Allergies – Because
many allergies stem from toxins and other
foreign agents in the body, zeolites can lesson
the risk or severity of allergies by trapping such
foreign agents.

4) Detoxification – Due to its
molecular structure, zeolite minerals are
capable of selectively attracting, binding, and
safely removing toxic particles, whether they
are heavy metals, radioactive particles, viruses,
or other dangerous substances. By removing
toxins from the system, zeolites can help the
body to defend itself while also increasing
strength, endurance, and stamina.

5) Antioxidant Function – Oxidative
stress can be increased when we are exposed to
pollution or chronic infections. This leads to

generation of free radicals, which are toxins generated inside the body instead of coming from environmental sources. If they are not neutralized, free radicals attack and damage healthy cells and their DNA, causing premature aging, immune dysfunction, and a myriad of dysfunctions and diseases. Zeolites can act as an antioxidant, countering free radicals and helping the body defend itself against this attack.

6) Antiviral Properties – Because of its net negative charge, zeolites can attract and bind to positively charged viral sub-particles. These are the particles that actually join together to form a new virus. By doing this, zeolites help to limit the proliferation of viruses which can then be safely removed from the body.

7) Immune-Stimulating Effects – Scientists believe that zeolites may be able to activate large groups of T-cells (the "killer" lymphocytes in the blood). In a study on patients being treated for immunodeficiency, six to eight weeks of zeolite supplementation was found to increase the blood counts of certain immune cells, enhancing the effect of the immune system.

8) Strengthen Immune System – Zeolites eliminate harmful substances, stop destructive attacks of free radicals, and find and bind pathogens in the circulatory system.

9) Normalize Blood Sugar – Glucose molecules carry a slight positive charge and as such have the capability of attaching themselves to the outside of a negatively charged zeolite particle. Through this passive mechanism, zeolites may help eliminate excess glucose and, as a result, help modulate blood sugar levels.

10) Sharpen Mental Acuity – Zeolites can protect the blood vessels and the tissues in the brain by trapping highly reactive free radicals and eliminating them from the system.

11) Protect Cardiovascular System – As free radicals travel through the blood, they set the stage for heart, vascular, myocardial, and cerebrovascular disease. Zeolites may help to trap free radicals along with environmental toxins, thereby preventing or limiting further damage.

12) Protect Membrane – Zeolites, in conjunction with the antioxidant network, protect vital cell membranes from degradation and weakening by the effects of the toxic substances.

13) Capture and Eliminate Toxins – Zeolite cavities are negatively charged compounds that attract and capture toxins and other harmful substances like free radicals in order to eliminate them. The elimination of these toxins allows the body's cells to stay functional and repair themselves when damaged.

14) Help Eliminate Heavy Metals – Heavy metals from environmental pollutants can accumulate in our body's organs and tissues. The most dangerous among them are lead, mercury, cadmium, and arsenic. They strain the ability of the liver to metabolize compounds for use in the body and eliminate toxic compounds. Zeolites can attract these compounds and eliminate them from the body.

15) Adaptogenic Properties – An adaptogen is something that reacts and interacts with other compounds, thereby helping the body "adapt" or normalize within its current health state. Zeolites are used by the body in a variety of ways, adapting to the body's needs and acting as an antioxidant, blood cleanser, cell strengthening mineral, and toxin remover.

You can find this supplement online and try it if it works for you. I think it might be VERY beneficial in expediting detoxing.

Olive leaf extract

The first time I heard about olive leaf extract was when I was suffering with seasonal allergies, and a friend offered me a tablespoon to see if it helps me. I didn't know much about it at that time, but she explained to me that it's anti-inflammatory, and can also help with my allergy symptoms. When I got home, I researched olive leaf extract thoroughly, and I realized that it's a useful find. I took one tablespoon a day for months, and it seemed to me that it helped me with my allergies. I would like to share the information I learned about this awesome extract with you. The following is an overview of an article that I found while researching, written by Julian Everson and titled "Unexpected Benefits of Olive Leaf Extract":

Scientists have isolated the unique molecule that provides olive oil with its multitude of health and life-extending benefits. Known as oleuropein, it is the polyphenol that can help lower bad cholesterol and blood pressure, prevent cancer, protect against oxidative damage, and help guard against cognitive decline. Oleuropein provides the distinctive tangy, pungent, almost bitter flavor found in high quality extra virgin olive oils. When oleuropein was given to animals with tumors, the tumors were completely regressed and disappeared in 9 to 12 days!

The olive tree (Olea europaea) produces oleuropein abundantly in its leaves as well as in the olive fruit itself. Special processing techniques now allow for the extraction of a stable, standardized form of oleuropein. This means that the consumers can have access to one of the most beneficial components of olive oil without the necessity of consuming excessive amounts of olive oil. Olive leaf extracts and their oleuropein constituents are best known for their blood pressure-lowering effects, but the latest studies reveal their health benefits extend well beyond that. Additional anti-inflammatory and antioxidant properties offer promise in fighting atherosclerosis, diabetes, cancer, neurodegenerative diseases, and even arthritis.

Animal studies demonstrate that olive leaf extracts lead to significant drops in elevated blood pressure. Remarkably, these effects are evident when supplementation occurs either before or after the animals develop hypertension. This means that the extracts have the ability to both prevent and treat high blood pressure. The drop in blood pressure is accompanied by reduced pressure in the heart's left ventricle. This results in improved blood flow to the heart's own coronary blood vessels. Additional human studies demonstrate the ability of olive leaf extracts to significantly reduce blood pressure measurements.

One particularly fascinating study was conducted among identical twins with borderline hypertension (blood pressure in the range of 120-139 mmHg over 80-89 mmHg). Studies of identical twins virtually eliminate genetic variations, which may impact study results. After 8 weeks of treatment, the placebo recipients showed no change in blood pressure from baseline, but patients supplemented with 1,000 mg/day of olive leaf extract dropped their pressures by a mean of 11 mmHg systolic and 4 mmHg diastolic. The supplemented patients experienced significant reductions in LDL cholesterol.

A human study measured olive leaf extract against captopril—one of the conventional drugs used for treating hypertension. In this study, patients with stage-1 hypertension (140-159 mmHg over 90-99 mmHg) took either 500 mg of olive leaf extract twice daily, or 12.5 mg of captopril twice daily, which was increased as needed, to 25 mg twice daily. After 8 weeks of treatment, both groups experienced a drop in the mean blood pressure from baseline (11.5 and 13.7 mmHg systolic; 4.8 and 6.4 mmHg diastolic, respectively), with no significant difference between the two groups.

In other words, the olive leaf extract performed as well as the prescription drug. A closer look in the laboratory reveals the reason for this equivalence. Although they utilize different mechanisms of action (oleuropein acts as a natural calcium channel blocker and captopril is a well-known ACE-inhibitor), both oleuropein and captopril function inside the vasculature to decrease the tension in the walls of blood vessels and promote widening of the vessels (vasodilation), ultimately lowering blood pressure. The proven blood pressure-lowering effects of olive leaf extracts are potent enough to warrant caution if you are taking prescription blood pressure drugs. If you are on blood pressure medication, it's essential that you speak to your doctor before starting supplementation.

Blood pressure is only one measure of cardiovascular health; arterial health is equally important. The endothelial cells that line arterial walls play a key role in maintaining blood flow and pressure as they also regulate the distribution of smooth muscle cells and sustain an even flow of blood through vessels. Endothelial dysfunction is one of the earliest stages in hardening of the arteries (atherosclerosis), which occurs when plaques build up in the arterial walls. These plaques eventually block blood flow and can trigger a heart attack or stroke.

Olive leaf extracts fight endothelial dysfunction at multiple levels. They also increase the production of nitric oxide, a signaling molecule that helps relax blood vessels. They reduce the production and activity of a class of molecules known as matrix metalloproteinases, or MMPs. Excessive MMP activity literally dissolves the gel-like matrix that holds cells together, making vessel linings increasingly vulnerable to plaque damage. They also help prevent the oxidation of LDL-cholesterol, which is one of the earliest events in developing atherosclerosis. Oxidized LDL triggers inflammation, further damaging arteries, and olive leaf extract has multi-targeted anti-inflammatory effects.

Polyphenol compounds found in olive leaves have been shown to directly help prevent the formation of arterial plaques (and thereby reduce the risk of heart attack and stroke) in two ways. Firstly, they reduce the production and activity of a series of "adhesion molecules." These substances cause white blood cells and platelets to stick to arterial walls, resulting in early plaque formation. Secondly, they reduce platelet aggregation (clumping) by multiple mechanisms, which reduces the risk that tiny clots will form at sites of plaque to produce a stroke or heart attack.

The diabetic (and pre-diabetic) state of chronic blood sugar elevation imposes substantial oxidative stress throughout the body, triggering inflammation and tissue damage that rapidly accelerates aging. Treatments for diabetes have two main goals: 1) lowering blood glucose to normal levels, and 2) limiting the damage done by the inevitable blood sugar spikes that still occur.

Olive leaf extracts are showing real promise in both of these areas. In animal and basic lab studies, olive leaf extracts and oleuropein have been found to lower blood sugar through several mechanisms. They slow the digestion of starches into simple sugars, slow absorption of those sugars from the intestine, and increase the uptake of glucose into tissues from the blood. They protect these tissues from the oxidant damage caused when glucose binds to proteins in the process called glycation. They also increase levels of other natural antioxidant systems in the body, broadening the degree of protection.

These mechanisms have directly observable benefits. Studies show that diabetic animals, supplemented with olive leaf extracts, experience significant reductions in blood sugar and cholesterol.

In a dramatic head-to-head study, diabetic rats were treated with either olive leaf extract or glyburide (Diabeta®), a common glucose-lowering drug. By the end of the study, the antidiabetic effects of the extract proved superior to those of the drug.

One intriguing study showed that when lab rats were fed a high-fat, high-carbohydrate diet, they developed all the signs of metabolic syndrome—excessive abdominal fat, hypertension, abnormal lipid profile, and impaired glucose tolerance. But when these animals were fed that unhealthy diet along with olive leaf extracts, virtually all of the metabolic abnormalities improved or, in some cases, normalized.

Human studies reveal that supplementing with 500 mg of olive leaf extract once daily resulted in significant reductions in hemoglobin A1c levels, the standard marker of long-term exposure to elevated blood sugar in diabetic people. Supplementation also lowered fasting plasma insulin levels, an important point because chronic insulin elevations may contribute to diabetics' higher cancer risks.

The Mediterranean diet is renowned for its ability to reduce the risk of cancer. While numerous aspects of the diet contribute to this risk reduction, there's growing evidence that olive oil, specifically its oleuropein content, are key components of the diet's anti-cancer effects. Studies show that oleuropein's antioxidant effects help it battle cancer formation at its earliest stages. Olive leaf extracts inhibit DNA damage from reactive oxygen species, which is the very first step in development of malignant cells. Once cells become cancerous, they rely on a host of chemical signaling factors that promote their growth and organization into tumors. Olive leaf compounds are known to inhibit growth factors and disrupt signalling pathways.

Oleuropein also suppresses an enzyme that cancer cells rely on to derive and store energy from dietary carbohydrates.

Oleuropein and olive leaf extracts have numerous other mechanisms of action against cancer. They help prevent inflammation, which is another major promoter of tumor growth. In breast cancer cells specifically, oleuropein reduces malignant cells' ability to respond to estrogen, the female hormone that many breast cancer cells depend on for their survival. Oleuropein inhibits the production of the "protein-melting" enzymes that cancer cells need in order to invade healthy tissues and metastasize to distant parts of the body.

These mechanisms have now been shown in laboratory and animal studies to reduce the rates of occurrence and subsequent development of a broad variety of cancers, including those of the brain, head and neck, breast, liver, bladder, prostate, and skin, as well as leukemia.

In one especially vivid study, mice with a high spontaneous cancer rate were orally supplemented with oleuropein. As a result, the tumors completely regressed and disappeared in 9 to 12 days. When the tumors were examined before they vanished, they were found to have a disordered, crumbly consistency, and no cancer cells remained alive within.

Olive extracts help protect the brain and central nervous system from the destruction brought on by strokes and age-related degenerative conditions such as Alzheimer's and Parkinson's diseases.They accomplish this by suppressing inflammation and reducing the damage done by oxidative stress. In acute brain injuries, such as those caused by a stroke or trauma, damaging processes such as oxidative stress occur within minutes of the original event and, ironically, are worsened by the return of normal blood flow to the area.

Researchers found a number of positive effects in animals that were pre-treated with olive leaf extract and then induced with a stroke. Compared to untreated animals, the treated animals experienced a sharp reduction in markers of oxidation and an increase in normal cellular antioxidant systems. Microscopic examination of brain tissue revealed a similar decline in injury to brain cells and up to a 55% decrease in the volume of dying brain tissue. Similar results are shown in experimental spinal cord injury in animals pretreated with oleuropein.

Olive leaf extracts offer similar protection for neurodegenerative diseases. Oxidative stress occurs more gradually in neurodegenerative diseases. However, the effects add up over a lifetime, producing inflammation and other changes that result in the accumulation of abnormal proteins that interfere with brain function and kill neurons. Olive leaf extracts help prevent these abnormal proteins from assembling into the neurofibrillary tangles seen in the brains of people with Alzheimer's and similar diseases.

Olive leaves and their extracts have long been used in the Mediterranean as folk remedies for arthritis. Now, scientific evidence has proven that olive leaf extracts can, in fact, interfere with the development of several different kinds of arthritis including gout, rheumatoid arthritis, and osteoarthritis.

Gout is caused by the accumulation of uric acid crystals in joints, which are the byproducts of impaired recycling of DNA and RNA in cells. In a mechanism identical to that of allopurinol (the gold standard drug therapy for gout), oleuropein prevents the buildup of uric acid by inhibiting xanthine oxidase, the enzyme responsible for converting DNA and RNA into uric acid.

Oleuropein has also been found to help prevent and treat symptoms of rheumatoid arthritis. When administered at the earliest sign of arthritis in animal models, oleuropein prevented symptoms from developing and also produced marked improvement in the microscopic appearance of joint tissue from affected animals. When administered after arthritis was fully developed, there was significant improvement in the inflammatory changes to joints, compared with untreated animals. Oleuropein had similar benefits on osteoarthritis. In animal models of this degenerative joint disease, olive leaf extract improved joint swelling, improved the microscopic appearance of joint tissue, and prevented the production of inflammatory cytokines.

The Mediterranean diet reduces your risk for virtually every condition associated with aging. Olive leaves contain higher amounts of oleuropein—a polyphenol with unique health-improving attributes. These extracts have been used in traditional medicine for centuries to improve age-related diseases. Convincing evidence now shows that oleuropein-rich olive leaf extracts help prevent many of the underlying factors leading to problems with health. Extra-virgin olive oil and olive leaf extract should be considered an important component of one's health and longevity program.

Wild oregano oil

Oregano oil is, as the name implies, oil from the oregano herb that is extracted by steam distillation. There are more than 40 varieties of the plant. According to *Alive*, the oil from Oreganum vulgare is believed to hold the most therapeutic benefit. Oregano is used for respiratory tract disorders such as coughs, asthma, croup, and bronchitis. It is also used for gastrointestinal (GI) disorders such as heartburn and bloating. Other uses include treating menstrual cramps, rheumatoid arthritis, urinary tract disorders including urinary tract infections (UTIs), headaches, and heart conditions.

I learned about the existence of wild oregano oil when I was looking at the health store for something that would replace my medication from allergies and was suggested to try it. I had a hard time breathing because of the seasonal allergies back then. But as soon as I took my first capsule of wild oregano oil, I found peace. I was able to breathe again within

20 minutes. I started using it instead of allergy pills when I needed some help (especially during seasonal allergies).

There is some evidence to suggest that it might be able to help stave off sickness in winter. Some natural health enthusiasts promote oregano oil as a means to fight cold and flus, keep your digestive tract healthy, and soothe skin problems. In addition to that, you may find some relief by adding a couple drops of oregano oil to a diffuser or vaporizer and inhaling it for a few minutes. Drinking a few drops of oil in juice or water may also provide some relief from a sore throat. The following is a summary of an article I found in my research, titled "Oil of Oregano Benefits: 11 Things To Know About Oregano Oil," written by Terri Coles and published in *Huffington Post*:

[Oregano oil] is also used for GI problems. Because there's some evidence that the oil of oregano has anti-fungal or anti-viral properties, it's thought to be helpful for some gastrointestinal issues.

Another small study showed that treatment with oregano oil may be useful for parasite infections, but further study is still needed.

It could have anti-fungal properties as well. Some studies have shown that in lab cultures, oregano oil puts up a strong fight against Candida albicans—the bacteria that causes the fungal infection, candida. Other research found it may have a similar effect against the mold fungis Aspergillus flavus and Aspergillus niger. However, similar studies haven't yet been conducted upon human subjects.

You can use it on your skin. It's thought that oregano oil is helpful for skin conditions like cold sores, muscle aches, nail fungus, joint pain, and dandruff. Try diluting it with a carrier oil like jojoba, sweet almond, or grapeseed, add 10 to 12 drops of oregano oil per ounce of carrier oil. However, don't use oregano oil on

broken or sensitive skin, as it can be
irritating. There is some anecdotal
evidence suggestions that it may be
effective for treatment of psoriasis, an
inflammatory skin condition, but there is
no published research yet.

It is also a natural insect repellent. The oil
of oregano contains many compounds,
and one of them is carvacrol — a natural
insect repellent. This compound is also
found in plants like mint and thyme. Try
putting a few drops of oil on the outdoor
furniture. Test first on an inconspicuous
area to make sure it doesn't stain, or
apply a dilution of it to unbroken skin
when heading outdoors.

It may help in the fight against antibiotic
resistance. Some people believe that we
can stave off antibiotic resistance by
turning to natural solutions like oregano
oil more often. One lab test in 2001 found
that oregano oil was effective in killing

staphylococcus bacteria. While another published laboratory study from the UK, found that it showed effectiveness against 25 different bacteria.

Keep in mind that pure oregano oil is very strong. If you are planning on using it topically, make sure you are using a diluted version so as to avoid irritation. Terri Coles suggests using one part oregano oil to three parts carrier oil. For internal ingestion, I preferred taking it in capsules, so that I wouldn't have to taste the stinging flavor in my mouth at its full strength.

Medicinal mushrooms

Reishi mushrooms

Reishi mushrooms are also called ganoderma. They are known for their reddish-brown color and their large, kidney-shaped top. While they aren't always easy to find, ganodermas are truly a hidden gem among mushrooms. Below is an overview of one of my favorite articles from HerbWisdom.com, titled "Ganoderma Benefits" that will help you understand why you might want to consider adding reishi mushrooms to your diet.

Reishi mushrooms are not often used in cooking because they are hard and have a bitter taste, although some people do use them in the same dishes that you might use shitake mushrooms. But you are unlikely to find them at your favorite market. They are mainly used for purely medicinal purposes and have a number of health benefits. In fact, it is known among practitioners of Chinese medicine as the "king of herbs."

All mushrooms are the "fruit" of fungi as well as the reproductive part. Reishi mushrooms can be found growing up from underground networks called mycelium near organic waste and logs, which are both a good nutrient source.

Given the right conditions, reishi can actually be cultivated and used in medicine. The Eastern world has been using reishi for thousands of years, particularly in China and Japan. Even the ancient kings and emperors drank reishi tea because it was believed that its properties encouraged vigor and long life. They also thought that the tea would increase their wisdom and happiness. The use of reishi has now reached the Western world where these days people are making elixirs from the mushroom for the purpose of promoting vitality and longevity. It is also used to treat certain medical conditions.

The benefits of ganoderma are so well known and proven that you can get them in forms that are much convenient than slicing them up and cooking them. You can buy them dried, in concentrated tablets, capsules, or even as an extract. In any of these forms, ganoderma can be used as a dietary supplement. Here is a list of the benefits that ganoderma have as a daily dietary supplement or in helping to treat certain medical conditions:

• **Antioxidants** – These mushrooms are very strong antioxidants. Antioxidants protect the body from the negative effects of free radicals that are formed inside the body by daily exposure to the sun, chemicals, and pollutants. Ganoderma are proven to boost the immune system, especially when taken with other antioxidant supplements.

• **Cancer Prevention** – It is believed that Ganoderma can suppress the growth of tumors in people who have cancer. It can reinforce the membranes in cancerous cells to keep the tumor from spreading. For this reason, they are often used in efforts to prevent cancers.

• **Respiratory Ailments** – Ganoderma are also beneficial for people suffering from asthma and other respiratory conditions because it seems to have a healing effect on the lungs. They are good for building respiratory strength and curbing a cough.

• **Anti-Inflammatory** – Ganoderma have anti-inflammatory properties and are, therefore, sometimes used for patients who have Alzheimer's and heart disease. This is based on the idea that inflammation plays a part in each of these conditions. The pain that accompanies other inflammatory conditions, like neuralgia and arthritis may also be lessened by ganoderma supplements.

• **Lowers Cholesterol** – As far as benefits for the heart, ganoderma can improve the flow of blood to the heart and reduce the amount of oxygen that the heart consumes. It can help to lower cholesterol and some of the ingredients may help combat high blood pressure.

So exactly what is it in ganoderma that give it so many health benefits? Scientists have learned that one active ingredient is polysaccharides, which contain beta glucan. Beta glucan is known for its ability to enhance the immune system—in fact, it is one of the strongest immune system supplements there is.

Another ingredient in ganoderma is triterpenes. The type found in ganoderma is a ganoderic acid that has been proven in studies to ease the symptoms of allergies by stopping the release of histamines. It can also improve the body's use of oxygen and help the liver function better.

I started using reishi mushrooms to help me alleviate the symptoms of allergies, and it seemed it was helping. I used reishi mushrooms for a while in my "tea." I would buy dried mushrooms, put them in a big pot and heat up the water (but not boil it). I would let it sit for 24 hours before I would drink four ounces of that "tea" in the evening and in the morning. You can easily make it in bulk and store it in the refrigerator for a couple of weeks. This tea is certainly beneficial for some ailments and can be a powerful aid in the process of detoxing and transitioning to a raw food lifestyle.

Chaga mushrooms

I have heard that chaga mushrooms help to open the "third eye," or to decalcify the pineal gland. I got really interested in this idea and started looking into it. What I learned is worth sharing, because it has a lot of beneficial medicinal qualities. Below is an exerpt from an article on UPChagaConnection.com titled "U.P. Chaga Facts & Benefits" that gives a great overview of this unique mushroom:

Rather than being soft like a mushroom, chaga is hard, almost as hard as wood. It is unique and is nothing like a common mushroom. In fact, chaga is most nutritionally dense among all tree growths. Known by the Siberians as the "Gift from God" and the "Mushroom of Immortality," this vibrant growth has been used by humans to support health for thousands of years. The Japanese call it "The Diamond of the Forest," while the Chinese deem it the "King of Plants." For the Chinese, that is saying a lot, since they have an immense history with countless plants. Now, you can get the great powerful secret of the Orient through North American Herb & Spice's wild chaga supplements. Despite this exceptional status, most Americans are unaware of it.

To survive in harsh climates, chaga concentrates natural compounds for its protection, which is why it is so powerful. To strengthen and heal the tree, it makes potent phytochemicals, including sterols, phenols, and enzymes. Researchers have inoculated sick trees with chaga to strengthen them. People benefit by consuming these forest-source phytochemicals and nutrients.

Chaga is so powerful, because it contains the nutrients—the force of actual trees. Because of their special, biologically potent substances, trees live long, far longer than herbs. Some trees live as long as 10,000 years or more. Concentrating this power, chaga contains numerous B vitamins, flavonoids, phenols, minerals, and enzymes. It is also one of the world's densest sources of pantothenic acid, and this vitamin is needed by the adrenal glands as well as digestive organs. It also contains riboflavin and niacin in significant amounts. In particular, it is highly rich in special phenols, which are pigment-like. These phenolic compounds are known as chromogenic complex. Chaga can be up to 30% chromogenic complex by weight. The chromogenic complex is highly protective for all tissues and is only found in chaga. In the cream base, this chromogenic complex is hightly protective of the skin. Rubbed on the skin, it even helps people develop a tan, because it contains the pigment melanin, the same pigment responsible for dark-colored skin.

Chaga contains wild-source minerals and is particularly high in copper, calcium, potassium, manganese, zinc, and iron. Yet, its most potent ingredient is a special substance known as superoxide dismutase (SOD). This is an enzyme with great potency. Its function is to halt oxidation, especially the toxicity of a free radical known as a singlet oxygen. This is the type of oxygen, which is responsible for oxidizing and damaging the tissues, which results in aging. It is the same oxygen which rusts a nail. SOD blocks this damage by quenching the singlet oxygen free radical.

The SOD content per gram of chaga is exceedingly high and accounts for many of its historical powers. Tests performed on North American Herb & Spice's wild chaga prove that it contains some 10,000 to 20,000 active SOD units per gram! This is an exceedingly high amount, far higher than that found even in typical

SOD pills. The typical SOD pill contains from 200 to 2,000 units per serving. So the difference is considerable. Plus, the type of SOD in pills is virtually impossible to absorb, while the wild chaga type is well-utilized by the body.

Chaga is a health food, which supports the entire system. The Siberians drink it daily. This is why they are long-living. A chaga drinker lives up to 85–100 years, while a non chaga-drinking person, the Inuit, lives only about 50 years. This proves that natural phytochemicals, the ones found in chaga, actually do make a difference. Yet, there is more traditional use that offers evidence.

Ancient Chinese regarded it as a longevity factor, which is why they deemed it the most complete of all growths. Japanese and Koreans use it regularly, and look how powerful they are today. In much of Siberia, Russia, and Eastern Europe it is an essential beverage. While the U.S. government restricts medical claims, here is what can be said: chaga has been used as an essential whole food supplement for many years by Russia's long-lived peasants, as well as long-lived villagers of Japan and Korea. These village people consume it as a daily beverage. They prefer it over common drinks such as tea and coffee. Because of its cleansing properties, in primitive Siberia the chaga drink was known as "soup water," although its taste is a pleasant combination of tea and coffee.

...Chaga was validated by Moscow's Medical Academy of Science, 1955, and was extensively used by the public. It is one of Russia's state secrets for power and strength, and was heavily used by champion Russian athletes, who defeated all others, including the best teams America could offer. So, the Russians,

Siberians, Poles, Romanians, Koreans, Japanese, and Chinese all use it.

...Here is what the Russians discovered. They found out that certain plants help your body fight the effects of stress and disease. They called these plants adaptogens. They discovered that chaga is the most potent adaptogen known. This is why it is the basis for the fight against premature aging and for prevention of serious diseases.

Since the 1950s the government of the Union of Soviet Socialist Republics (USSR), in conjunction with approximately 1,200 prominent scientists, conducted over 3,000 experiments involving 500,000 people to study the effects of adaptogens. An adaptogen is a substance which modifies the human body's response to stress. The results of these studies were a protected Soviet secret for 40 years. The Soviet government commanded athletes, astronauts, and other Soviet elites to take adaptogens on a daily basis to improve physical and mental work capacity. One of these adaptogens was chaga. In fact, of all these adaptogens, chaga was found to be the most powerful. It is now believed that up to 80% of all diseases are mainly due to stress.

Be sure to get the original chaga, which is truly wild and free of all chemicals and solvents. I would recommend to get wild-harvested chaga. A simple cup or two of this tea has a dramatic effect—and all without any stimulants. No matter which chaga product you take, you can feel the difference immediately. Experience the immense power of wild birch tree power. This is the energy and power of the wild-source enzymes, notably SOD, peroxidase, and nucleases, as well as wild sterols, phenols, B vitamins, minerals, and much more.

Here are the benefits of chaga mushrooms that David Wolfe cited:

- Chaga mushrooms, when consumed on a regular basis, can slow ageing, improve health and provide anti-aging benefits.

- Various studies and researches have found out that consumption of Chaga mushrooms offers protection against damage of an oxidative kind to the human lymphocytes DNA.

- Because of immuno stimulation, Chaga mushrooms also fight against cancerous growths and cancer cells.

- The presence of betulinic acid in Chaga mushrooms or betulin, inhibits the growth of tumors and kills off tumor tissues as well as tumor cells. So if you suffer from tumors, it is beneficial to consume Chaga mushrooms.

- Chaga mushrooms are your safest bets when it comes to creating general feelings of well-being, increasing life span, delaying the signs of ageing, preventing aging and derailing cancer cells.

- It can help to heal injuries and rashes when applied on the skin.

- When consumed orally in the form of tea or powder or when inhaled in the form of smoke, it helps to boost the immune system, promote longevity, preserve youth, and it may be regarded as the elusive fountain of youth.

- Since 16th century, ancient eastern Europeans have been using Chaga mushrooms to treat gastritis, tuberculosis, ulcers, and cancers of different kinds and to promote general health.

- It can repair damaged DNA by producing interferons and it can also inhibit oxidation caused by free radicals. It can decrease hypoxia in organisms and maximize the stability of the body. The metabolic functions of the cell are rectified as well through consumption of Chaga mushrooms.

- Chaga mushrooms also possess anti-cancer properties in the form of betulinic acid and betulin.
- Chaga mushrooms provide an anti-inflammatory effect, stimulate metabolism in brain tissues, prevent cancerous growths and boost life energy or "chi."
- It can effectively help you get rid of kidney stones and sand.
- It also helps to combat the hormonal imbalance, HIV, diabetes, and immune deficiencies.

Shitake mushrooms

In one of his books, David Wolfe mentions medicinal mushrooms, and states that none of the other mushrooms should be eaten unless they are medicinal. All the other mushrooms are simple fungus that won't do any good for your internal organs (especially if you have problems with candida). Provided mushrooms grow and act like a sponge, they suck all the toxic matter onto themselves. For example, to clear the environment from radiation, it is good to use mushrooms that absorb all the toxic matter. David Wolfe mentions all the medicinal mushrooms and why using them is so beneficial. As reported by The Washingtonian:

> "Shiitake mushrooms are a great addition to anyone's diet and are mainly known for their immune system support," says dietitian Kait Fortunato. They contain lentinan, which makes our immune system strong, helping to fight off disease and infection. The American Cancer Society says that lentinan is believed to stop or slow tumor growth, though it also notes that more clinical trials are needed to understand the mushrooms' effectiveness.

According to Epicurist.com, Shiitake mushrooms have brown, slightly convex caps that range in diameter from about two to four inches in diameter. They belong to the basidiomycete family of fungi. Until the early 1990's, they were widely known by their scientific genus-species name of "Lentinus edodes." However, during the late 1980's and early 1990's this genus-species name for shiitake mushrooms was largely phased out and replaced by a new genus-species name, Lentinula edodes.

The common name for this mushroom, "shiitake," comes from the Japanese language. "Shii" in Japanese refers to wood belonging to the Pasania species of tree on which shiitake mushrooms naturally grow. "Take" simply translates as "mushroom." You may sometimes also hear shiitake mushroom being referred to as the "Black Forest mushroom," and they do indeed grow naturally in that German mountain range.

Acting as a symbol of longevity in Asia because of their health-promoting properties, shiitake mushrooms have been used medicinally by the Chinese for more than

545

6,000 years. More recently, their rich, smoky flavor has endeared them to the American taste buds.

Although immune system support has often received much of the spotlight in shiitake mushroom research, recent study results involving support of the cardiovascular system have also caught the attention of many researchers. In particular, recent studies have shown the ability of shiitake mushrooms to help protect us against cardiovascular diseases (including atherosclerosis) by preventing too much immune cell binding to the lining of our blood vessels.

As Tim Layman explains in his book, *Death Was Not An Option!*: "In order for immune cells and other materials to bind onto our blood vessel linings, certain protein molecules—called adhesion molecules—must be produced and sent into action. By helping to block the adhesion molecule production process, substances in shiitake mushrooms can help protect our blood vessels. The adhesion molecule production that is partially blocked by shiitake mushroom components includes the adhesion molecules ICAM-1, VCAM-1, and E-selectin."

EnigmaticHealing.com states that shiitake mushrooms have a long history as an iron-rich food. Recent studies have hinted that shiitake mushrooms may have an even better bioavailability than nutritionists first beleved. A lab study featuring female rats found that dried shiitake mushrooms contain bio-available iron that is nearly identical to supplemental iron. For those who prefer to get iron from non-animal products, the quality of iron in shiitake mushrooms is very promising.

Tim Layman supports the nutritional value of shiitake mushrooms further: "People do not usually consider including mushrooms as part of their meals because of their nutritional content. However, shiitake mushrooms are rich in B vitamins—they are an excellent source of pantothenic acid, a very good source of vitamin B2, a good source of vitamin B6, niacin, choline, and folate. Additionally, they are concentrated in minerals, being an excellent source of selenium and copper, a very good source of zinc, and a good source of manganese. They are also a good source of vitamin D (in the D2 form) and dietary fiber. They also provide a wide variety of unique phytonutrients."

No health benefit of the shiitake mushroom is better documented than its powerful ability to support the immune system. Many scientific studies have demonstrated that whole shiitake mushrooms can stabilize the immune system, keeping overactive immune systems at bay.

Some studies even point to shiitake mushrooms as being able to stimulate immune system responses in certain cases. What we can learn from both segments of scientific study is that shiitake mushrooms can either stimulate or suppress the immune system as needed, making these mushrooms a valuable addition to a healthy diet.

The following excerpt from *Death Was Not An Option!* offers an in-depth exploration of how shiitake mushrooms provide particular benefit to the immune system:

One especially interesting area of immune system support involves the impact of shiitake mushrooms on immune cells called macrophages. Among their many important activities, macrophage cells are responsible for identifying and clearing potentially cancerous cells from the body. In order to carry out this task, they need to be "activated" in a particular way. In more scientific terms, their activated phenotype needs to reflect a higher level of interleukin 1-beta and tumor necrosis factor alpha, and a lower level of interleukin 10. Shiitake mushrooms are able to help macrophage cells achieve this activated profile so that they can do a better job clearing potentially cancerous cells. Researchers refer to this result as an "anti-cancer immunity" that is enhanced by shiitake mushroom intake.

The most famous immune-supportive components in shiitake mushrooms are its polysaccharides. Polysaccharides are large-sized carbohydrate molecules composed of many different sugars arranged in chains and branches. Although many fungi are well-known for their polysaccharides, no single fungus has been more carefully studied than the shiitake mushroom. We know that this fungus is unique in its variety of polysaccharides, and especially its polysaccharide glucans. (Glucans are polysaccharides in which all of the sugar components involve the simple sugar glucose.) Among the glucans contained in shiitake mushroom are alpha-1,6 glucan, alpha-1,4 glucan, beta-1,3 glucan, beta-1,6 glucan, 1,4-D-glucans, 1,6-D-glucans, glucan phosphate, laminarin, and lentinan.

Shiitake mushrooms also contain some important non-glucan polysaccharides, including fucoidans and galactomannins. The immune-related effects of polysaccharides in shiitake mushrooms have been studied on laboratory animals under a wide variety of circumstances, including exercise stress, exposure to inflammation-producing toxins, radiation exposure, and immunodeficiency. Under all of these circumstances, the polysaccharides in shiitake mushrooms have been shown to lessen problems. There is also some evidence that the polysaccharides in shiitake mushrooms can help lower total cholesterol levels.

The cardiovascular benefits of shiitake mushrooms have been documented in three basic areas of research. The first of these areas is cholesterol reduction. D-Eritadenine (also called lentinacin, or lentsine, and sometimes abbreviated as DEA) is one of the most unusual naturally occurring nutrients in shiitake mushrooms that has repeatedly been shown to help lower total blood cholesterol. This nutrient is actually derived from adenine—one of the building blocks (nucleotides) in the mushroom's genetic material (DNA). The beta-glucans in shiitake mushrooms are also very likely to contribute to its cholesterol-lowering impact.

Another basic area of cardiovascular support involves the interaction between our cardiovascular system and our immune system. Recent studies have shown that shiitake mushrooms can help protect us against cardiovascular diseases (including atherosclerosis) by preventing too much immune cell binding to the lining of our blood vessels. In order for immune cells and other materials to bind onto our blood vessel linings, certain protein molecules—called adhesion molecules—must be produced and sent into action.

By helping to block the adhesion molecule production process, substances in shiitake mushrooms can help protect our blood vessels. (The adhesion molecule production, which is partially blocked by shiitake mushroom components, includes the adhesion molecules ICAM-1, VCAM-1, and E-selectin.)

A final basic area of cardiovascular benefits involves antioxidant support. Chronic oxidative stress in our cardiovascular system (ongoing, oxygen-based damage to our blood vessel linings) is a critical factor in the development of clogged arteries (atherosclerosis) and other blood vessel problems. One of the best ways for us to reduce our risk of chronic oxidative stress is consumption of a diet that is rich in antioxidant nutrients.

Shiitake mushrooms are a very good source of three key antioxidant minerals such as manganese, selenium, and zinc.

They also contain some unusual phytonutrient antioxidants. One of the best studied is ergothioneine (ET). This unique antioxidant is derived from the amino acid histidine, although it is unusual since it contains a sulfur group of molecules that are not present in histidine itself.

In studies on ET and our cells' oxidative stress levels, one fascinating finding has been the special benefits of ET for cell components called mitochondria. Mitochondria use oxygen to produce energy for the cell. The heart cells have greater concentrations of mitochondria than most other cell types in the body. For this reason, researchers believe that ET may be one of the key nutrients from shiitake mushrooms that provide us with cardiovascular support.

Most of the research on shiitake mushrooms and cancer has been

conducted on laboratory animals or on
individual cells in a laboratory setting and
has involved mushroom extracts rather
than whole mushrooms in eatable food
form. For this reason, our understanding
of the anti-cancer benefits of shiitake
mushrooms as a whole, natural food is
still preliminary. But based on research to
date, we believe that adding shiitake
mushrooms to your diet is likely to offer
you anti-cancer benefits, especially with
respect to prevention of prostate cancer,
breast cancer, and colon cancer.

Medicinal extracts from shiitake
mushrooms have been studied much
more extensively than the mushroom as
food itself. In laboratory animal
experiments, numerous components of
shiitake mushrooms have been shown to
help block tumor growth, sometimes by
triggering programmed cell death
(apoptosis) in the cancer cells. These
components have been collectively

referred to as "anti-tumor mycochemicals" provided by shiitake mushrooms. Researchers have speculated that more than a 100 different types of compounds in shiitake mushrooms may work together to accomplish these anti-tumor results. While the unique polysaccharides in shiitake mushrooms were first thought to be its primary anti-cancer compounds, scientists are now convinced that shiitake provides many non-polysaccharide substances that have anti-tumor effects.

The special combination of antioxidants found in shiitake mushrooms, together with their highly flexible support for immune system function, make them a natural candidate for providing us with protection from a variety of problems involving oxidative stress and immune function. This includes rheumatoid arthritis (RA), an area that has begun to interest shiitake mushroom researchers. Although research in this area is preliminary, it is expected to see large-scale human studies confirming the benefits of shiitake mushrooms for prevention of RA.

Medicinal extracts from shiitake mushrooms have had well-documented effects on a variety of micro-organisms, including bacteria, fungi, and viruses (including human immunodeficiency virus-1, or HIV-1). While we have yet to see large-scale human studies on the whole food intake of shiitake mushrooms and decreased susceptibility to colds, flu or other problems related to unwanted activity of micro-organisms, this is a very likely area for future food research and discovery of health benefits.

Shiitake mushrooms are undoubtedly a super food, but you shouldn't eat a whole plate of this mushrooms—especially raw. If you want to consume them in raw state, I believe that half of a mushroom cut in your salad would be enough. If you are a vegan, but are not 100% raw, then you can sauté mushrooms (no more than three or four of them) for seven minutes. But you should never eat raw shiitake mushrooms in high amounts, as your body will not react well. It might lead to upset stomach and diarrhea. Be careful with super foods and do not overdo them.

Jiaogulan tea

Jiaogulan is not yet a common element of the Western diet, but it has a long history in the East. This plant is a climbing vine that can be found in Korea, Japan, and China. It's closely related to familiar grocery staples such as pumpkins, cucumbers, and watermelons. Jiaogulan tea is a popular drink, and there are a range of health benefits to be had from adding Jiaogulan to your diet (although it should be mentioned that the effects during pregnancy and breastfeeding have not been studied). Some of the benefits of Jiaogulan tea include its ability to lower cholesterol, protect against arteriosclerosis, slow down signs of aging, build immunity, and provide a shield against cancer.

The excerpt below from Herbs4Cure.com does a great job of explaining the health benefits of Jiaogulan:

Scientific research studies in China have shown that Jiaogulan (Jiao Gu Lan) decreases cholesterol by improving the liver's ability to send sugar and carbohydrates to the muscles for conversion into energy, instead of turning the sugar into triglycerides, which the body stores as fat. It lowers LDL's (bad cholesterol) while raising HDL's (good cholesterol). It improves fat metabolism, reduces blood fat levels and depresses lipid peroxide and fat sediment in the blood vessels.

While it is great for rectifying high cholesterol and obesity problems, it can also improve and strengthen the digestion. This allows an underweight person to increase absorption of nutrients and gain weight in the form of lean muscle mass. This regulatory effect on bodily functions is the hallmark of an adaptogen.

Jiaogulan prevents cells from turning cancerous and also inhibits the growth of tumors already formed by stimulating the body's immune system cells. Cancer patients given Jiaogulan have shown marked improvement in white blood cell count antibody levels, and raised T and B lymphocyte levels. It has been shown that Jiaogulan has activity against esophagal, lung, breast, uterus, prostate, brain, kidney, thymus, and skin cancer.

Jiaogulan is one of the best broad-spectrum adaptogenic herbs known, containing polysaccharides, amino acids, vitamins, minerals, flavones, saponins and many essential trace elements. It is very safe for long-term use and is highly effective in reducing the side-effects of radiation and chemotherapy by boosting the immune system.

Athletes use Jiaogulan to enhance their performance because it enhances the heart pumping function, improving contraction of the heart muscle. The most pronounced benefits are increased endurance during strong physical activity, and more rapid recovery afterwards.

Jiaogulan contains 84 beneficial saponins—three times more than ginseng—yet it has no side-effects. Due to its significantly higher quantity of beneficial saponins, it has been widely studied and used worldwide, even for patients recovering from exposure to ultraviolet, beta and gamma-rays. It also dramatically reduces cholesterol levels, normalizes blood pressure, protects the heart, and increases fat metabolism.

Over 300 scientific research findings back up nearly every claim for Jiaogulan (also known as Gynostemma pentaphyllum). Jiaogulan is a superb immune-enhancer and an antioxidant for all ages.

Jiaogulan dramatically decreases the chances of a stroke by inhibiting blood platelets from "sticking together," which prevents a stroke-inducing blood clot from forming. This same action prevents artery clogging, reducing risk of a heart attack.

In China, doctors prescribe daily doses of Jiaogulan for patients recovering from heart and brain surgery, because the herb supports the immune system, aiding in a quicker and more effective recovery. Patients undergoing cancer therapies such as radiation and chemotherapy receive Jiaogulan as well. Research has also shown that Jiaogulan can increase the white blood cell count, which strengthens resistance, thus improving the patients' ability to recover.

Biochemist Subbuti Dharmenanda says that signs of aging are avoidable if you can tame the free radicals that cause them. "If free radicals aren't shut down, they cause everything from cataracts to cancer." But, studies show that taking just 40 mg of jiaogulan daily triples production of superoxide dismutase—a chemical that neutralizes free radicals by 21%.

Jiaogulan tea has been traditionally used as a remedy for bronchitis. In one study, the effectiveness rate of using jiaogulan tea to treat chronic bronchitis was 93%.

Jiaogulan has a bi-phasic action on the central nervous system, calming the nerves when irritated and exciting them when depressed. This is why Jiaogulan is known as an adaptogen. The increased balance affects other systems of the body as it helps in normalizing the balance between other organs' functions, thereby bolstering stability of the body as a whole. This results in better brain function, increased endurance, and resistance to illness and injury.

Antioxidants are an important factor in treating cancer, liver disease, diabetes, arteriosclerosis, arthritis inflammation and even the aging process. Jiaogulan has been proven in many studies to have a powerful antioxidant effect, by protecting the body from free radical damage.

Jiaogulan dramatically decreases the chances of a stroke by inhibiting blood platelets from "sticking together," which prevents the formation of stroke-inducing blood clots. This same action prevents artery clogging, thereby reducing risk of a heart attack. Also, studies show that in as little as two weeks, a small dose of Jiaogulan taken daily, lowers high blood pressure to a normal range. By increasing production of nitric oxide—a chemical that relaxes blood vessel walls—the herb effectively reduces the blood pressure. In addition, it reduces cholesterol by about 25%.

Vitamins

I believe that we don't need supplements to maintain a balanced and healthy life style. However, I used to have a different opinion before I started my journey to infinite health. I used to take all those fancy multi-vitamins that are advertised everywhere. I felt like I needed calcium and all sorts of other fancy things I was able to put my hands on. But, when I started researching the subject, I was deeply distraught when I uncovered my own ignorance. I believe that the majority of the population is on the same page, right where I used to be. Here's what I've learned through my research and experience.

First of all, if we do decide to take vitamins, we have to make sure that they are bio-available to us. If vitamins are not bio-available, our bodies will recognize them as non-organic, toxic, and inert matter. Even though we would feel some short-lived semi-effects from the non-bio-available vitamins (because they are stimulants), they will damage

566

our system in the long run. In order to be bio-available, vitamins have to be either raw or chelated.

Just to clarify, chelated vitamins will cost you roughly $200 or more per month, which not many people can afford. All over-the-counter versions of regular, cheap vitamins that the majority of people use are not chelated. That means they are not bio-available and, therefore, are toxic. So, your best bet would be to get all of your vitamins from raw fruits and veggies.

If you do want to take supplements, I would suggest using alternatives. For example, if you are looking for vitamin C, I recommend that you start experimenting. Move away from synthetic forms of vitamin C or ascorbic acid and look at powdered plants that are really high in vitamin C. For example, you can choose acerola cherry. This tropical berry is really high in vitamin C and is sold in dried powder form.

That's a really great way to naturally get lots of vitamin C with all the co-factors. Vitamin C needs co-factors like rutin and bioflavonoids that are all naturally present in powdered acerola cherry. You can either take it supplementally, or you can add it into your smoothies. You can literally put it in your glass of water and drink it as is.

The more I researched the supplements, the more I realized that most of them are useless at the very least—and toxic at most. I was taking vitamin C in the form of powder from Camu Camu berry, and discarded all the other "vitamins" that I had on my shelf. That was at the very beginning of my transition to raw foods. Once I switched to a 100% fruitarian diet, I quit supplements altogether, because I didn't feel the need for them any longer.

Calcium supplements

In an interview with *Editorial Today*, David Wolfe discussed calcium supplements at length. The following is a summary of his insights:

> Calcium does not build bones. This is one of the biggest misconceptions ever. Silicon and magnesium are the keys to increasing bone density. So, stop taking calcium and start taking silicon and magnesium to increase your bone density. Foods that contain silicon include: Bell peppers, green leafy vegetables, whole grains (sprouted), alfalfa, beets, nettles, hemp leaf and horsetail. Magnesium is found in: Nuts such as cashews, almonds, and macadamia. Also foods like avocados, spinach, and green leafy vegetables are enriched with magnesium.
>
> If you take calcium supplements, be aware that it turns out that all the calcium

supplements are contaminated with calcium forming organisms—they look like microscopic snails with shell on their backs that protects them—that once in our bodies, would re-produce geometrically in our system and cause inflammation, and block the arteries. They build like a coral reef and wherever they are—we have a problem: if it's in the heart—we get a heart attack, if it's in the joints—we get arthritis, if in the lungs— we get emphysema, if it gets in kidneys— we get kidney stones. So, you literally can become calcified, or turn into stone.

But let's get on to silicon because this is the mineral that is difficult to get in today's diet. Silicon is a mineral. You get it in the skin of cucumbers. It's in the skin of bell peppers. It's in the skin of tomatoes. It's in certain special herbs (horse tail, nettle, and oat straw), which you can drink as a tea or take it in supplemental form and you will notice that it helps with your bone density.

How does silicon increase calcium? I mean that doesn't make sense, right? It's because our theory of minerals is incorrect. Our atomic theory is incorrect. And that is if you eat silicon rich food, your body, through the power of enzymes transmutates it into calcium, i.e., turns the silicon into calcium. That was discovered by a great French researcher by the name of Louis Curvan, a Nobel prize nominee, who wrote five books and 5,000 pages of research on just this particular subject: how silicon and calcium are related to each other. It was very well honored in France and he is very intimately entwined in the science of what's going on in France; but because of the language barrier his research really never made it to the English-speaking nations.

...This is so engrained in our minds about calcium that if you are confused about this, get on the Internet and research exactly who is getting the results of remineralizing their bones and you'll find that it's people who are not taking these forms of calcium that are toxic, which is the oyster shell calcium, and to some degree even coral calcium. You have to make sure we get the right nutrition to build strong bones.

...The other side of the equation is we've got to make sure we are doing things that aren't hurting our bones. Eating lots of refined sugar is one of the worse things we can do to our overall health or our teeth (which are living bones), and to the density of our bones because when we take in lots of refined sugar, our body has to use calcium, it has to pull calcium out of the bones to buffer or neutralize the intense acidity of the sugar. Calcium is highly alkaline. Our bones are alkaline and, therefore, alkaline minerals are used whenever we're exposed to really strong acids. Sugar is a very strong acid. I mean, you know, that people dissolve the corrosion on their battery terminals of the bus by dumping soda pop onto it because that sugar just dissolves and the phosphoric acid just dissolves all the corrosion right on the battery terminal. I mean, you don't want to be putting that in your body. That's dangerous.

...The nations that consume the most calcium, the United States, Canada and the "Scandinavian countries, have the worst osteoporosis and that's because our theory of mineralization or our theory of nutrition is incorrect. The general theory is that a hundred years ago they started looking at people's bones. They found out that, "oh my god; these bones are made out of calcium." When people don't have enough bone density the thought is, "oh they just have to eat more calcium because that's what builds bones."

...Calcium does not build bones and that is one of the biggest misconceptions ever and it actually goes to the real core of our problems with science. And that is the human body is a complex biological machine of an unbelievable mystery. And there is strong evidence that indicates that if you eat some of the calcium, let's say it's calcium from coral, for example, or oyster shell calcium, then it is almost impossible to get that stuff into your bones to increase bone density. The amount of increasing bone density, at best, is 1 or 2%. It is not good enough.

So, do we need to eat more calcium to build more calcium? NO! If you are a raw foodist, you have nothing to worry about: you are already getting enough nutrition to build your calcium. (Of course, the side effects mentioned above are enough to make calcium supplements not worth the effort altogether.) The only attention you have to put on is silicon and magnesium.

Silicon is found particularly in mature grass right before it flowers. Young wild plants have high silicon for bone density, and mature wild plants like dandelion have high calcium. Grasses in nature do the reverse: they have calcium that they convert into silicon as they mature. Most weeds take silicon and convert it into calcium. Mature grass or young sprouted plants are high in silicon, and that's what we need to build calcium. Horsetail extract is high in silicon as well as bamboo leaf, bamboo sap, hemp leaf, oat straw, and nettles (highest content of silicon and iron). Raw plantian is high in magnesium. Pumpkin seeds are also high in magnesium, as well as spinach, parsley, garlic, chives, and coconut meat.

D3 vitamin

Much of the interest in vitamin D stems from the fact that it's found throughout the body in over 600 receptor sites, including the brain and the heart. Because vitamin D receptors are so prevalent in the body, ongoing research has been increased on vitamin D, and seemingly every day, new studies are released that tout the health benefits of vitamin D consumption.

Recent research has shown that vitamin D supports immune health by helping to regulate the immune system. The brain is home to dozens of vitamin D receptor sites, and vitamin D has been proven to enhance memory and concentration. It also supports healthy digestion, since receptor sites are found from the mouth all the way through the intestines. Healthy vitamin D levels support two increasing areas of concern—breast health for women and prostate health for men. The BarefootAndHealthy.com article outlined below by Chris D. Meletis, ND, provides a great overview of vitamin D:

> This vitamin is unique because cholecalciferol (Vitamin D3) is a vitamin derived from 7-dehyrocholesterol. Vitamin D3 acquires hormone-like actions when cholecalciferol (Vitamin D3) is converted to 1,25-dihydroxy Vitamin D3 (Calcitriol) by the liver and kidneys. As a hormone, Calcitriol controls phosphorus, calcium, and bone metabolism and neuromuscular function. Vitamin D3 is the only vitamin the body can manufacture from sunlight (UVB). Yet, with today's indoor living and the extensive use of sunscreens due to concern about skin cancer, we are now a society with millions of individuals deficient in life-sustaining, bone building and immune modulating 1,25-dihydroxy Vitamin D3.

...For more than a century, scientists have recognized that Vitamin D3 is involved in bone health. Research has continued to accumulate, documenting Calcitriol's role in the reduction of the risk of fractures to a significant degree. The latest research, however, shows that 1,25-dihyroxy Vitamin D3 *deficiency* is linked to a surprising number of other health conditions such as depression, back pain, cancer, both insulin resistance and pre-eclampsia and insulin resistance during pregnancy, high blood pressure, impaired immunity, and macular degeneration. [I've seen studies that also connect vitamin D3 to fibromyalgia, diabetes, multiple sclerosis, and rheumatoid arthritis. Most recently, low Vitamin D3 levels have been linked to an increased prevalence of early, age-related, macular degeneration.]

The Recommended Daily Intake (RDI) of Vitamin D3 is set so low that those mature individuals who consume this small amount (400 to 600 International Unites (I.U.'s)) are still likely to be deficient if they live north of the Tropic of Cancer or south of the Tropic of Capricorn. In fact, researchers have discovered that the RDI, which was considered adequate to prevent osteomalacia (a painful bone disease) or rickets, is not high enough to protect against the majority of diseases linked to 1,25-dihyroxy Vitamin D3 deficiency. For example, an analysis of the medical literature found that at least 1,000 to 2,000 IU of Vitamin D3 per day is necessary to reduce the risk of colorectal cancer and that lower doses of Vitamin D3 did not have the same protective effect.

Vitamin D3 deficiency is common in older adults and has been associated with psychiatric and neurological disorders. For example, in one study of 80 older adults (40 with mild Alzheimer's disease and 40 nondemented persons), Vitamin D3 deficiency was associated with low mood and with impairment on two of four measures of cognitive performance.

...Scientists are developing a greater appreciation for Vitamin D3's ability to improve cognition. In a recent study, Vitamin D3 deficient subjects scored worse on mental function tests compared to individuals who had higher levels of the Vitamin.

One of the best known and long-established benefits of vitamin D3 is its ability to improve bone health and the health of the musculoskeletal system. It is well-documented that vitamin D3 deficiency causes osteopenia, precipitates and exacerbates osteoporosis, causes a painful bone disease known as osteomalacia, and exacerbates muscle weakness, which increases the risk of falls and fractures. Lack of vitamin D3 may alter the regulatory mechanisms of parathyroid hormone (PTH) and cause a secondary hyperparathyroidism that increases the risk of osteoporosis and fractures. Musculoskeletal disorders have been linked to vitamin D3 deficiency in a number of studies. Some of these studies have explored the role that low vitamin D3 levels play in the development of chronic low back pain in women.

If you do choose to use a vitamin D3 supplement, please make sure that it's raw vegan with no additives. The best raw D3 vitamin I found is made by Vitamin Code—and it's not that expensive, so anyone can afford it.

Of course, the best way to get your vitamin D is by being outside and by getting enough sun. However, people are afraid of getting skin cancer, and therefore, they use a lot of sunblock. This is an interesting issue: on one hand, you don't have to be afraid of the sun, provided you are not toxic. But if you are toxic, then you will sweat out these toxins on to the surface of your skin and—quite literally— burn them onto the surface of your skin, which might cause cancer. If your system is clean, then it's a good idea to be exposed to the sun as much as possible. Despite what society may tell you, it will not cause aging or cancer.

I am warning again: do not overexpose yourself to too much sun without protection if you are just at the beginning of your transition to raw vegan foods, and if you are toxic! When I mention protection, I mean clothes that will create a barrier from the sun. I am not talking about sunblocks that cause cancer by themselves: no matter how "healthy" they claim to be, sunblock is a cream filled with toxins that you smear all over your body. I have a rule of thumb: what you can't eat, don't put on your skin, because you absorb everything you apply onto it. So, if you think it's crazy to put that sunblock on your plate and eat, I would say it's not the best idea to put it on your body and marinate yourself in those toxins. Instead, use coconut oil or hemp oil, as these are mild sun-blockers.

I think it's important to help your body at the very beginning of transitioning into raw foods and give it a little extra nutrition. I also read that vitamin D3 (or rather, the D3 hormone) helps with allergies, and that was one of the reasons I started taking it. Once you are adjusted to raw vegan foods, it would be a good time to let go of supplements (and never look back). It's best to never use any supplement for a prolonged period of time: it's just a crutch for a short period of time to re-balance your system.

Healthy sources of iron

The best organic iron sources are organically grown green leafy vegetables, raw spinach (raw is best since cooked spinach has some oxalic acid), parsley, watercress, sprouts, war squash, Swiss chard, dandelion and mustard greens, green cabbage, leeks, sorrel, Bibb lettuce, green lettuce, the skins of unwaxed cucumbers, avocado, horseradish, beet greens, artichokes, asparagus, carrots, tomatoes, beets, black radish, and pumpkin.

Many fresh, organically grown fruits and their juices have a high content of organic iron. Leading the list are blackberries, raspberries, blueberries, gooseberries, and grapes, cherries, oranges, peaches, strawberries and pears. Natural sun-dried fruits are high in iron. Apricots are the highest, followed by black figs, prunes, peaches, dates, and raisins.

Many other foods have a high content of iron: some of those include blackstrap and Barbados molasses, raw and unsalted sesame, pumpkin seeds, sunflower seeds, sprouted beans of all kinds (pinto, kidney, lima, lentils, garbanzos), peas and other raw and unsalted nuts.

All these foods will have a higher content of iron if grown organically with no chemical fertilizers and absolutely no poisonous sprays. And remember: your body needs ORGANIC IRON—not the iron that comes from inorganic sources (like non-chelated supplements).

Can our bodies get iron from water? You often hear about a certain well or spring containing large amounts of iron. Some waters do contain inorganic iron. But your body can't use this inorganic inert iron—in fact, this iron is dangerous to your body. It can cause all kinds of stones to form in your vital organs, cement your joints, and could turn your blood vessels to stone. No matter what, the best thing is to stay away from inorganic minerals!

Enzymes: Systemic and digestive

Whether breaking down foods or healing from injury, nearly every process the human body performs involves chemical reactions. Enzymes are proteins that act as the catalysts for these chemical reactions. Every cell in the body uses enzymes for building, maintenance, and repair.

The human body produces many enzymes on its own; however, natural production of enzymes begins to decline as early as the age of 25. Joint pain, circulatory problems, slower healing, and an increase in the incidence of disease are all too common with people who are enzyme deficient and suffering the effects of aging. Enzymes fall into three main categories: food enzymes, digestive enzymes, and systemic enzymes.

Food enzymes are found naturally in raw food. They help with joint health, arterial health, and the immune system. You can increase your intake of these enzymes by eating a healthy organic diet—rich in fruits and vegetables—and avoiding processed foods. You can also take it one step further by opting for an entirely raw vegan diet. Raw food is meant to decompose, so it essentially digests itself without your body wasting its energy.

Digestive enzymes, as their name implies, aid in the digestive process. They help the body break down fiber (cellulase), protein (protease), carbohydrates (amylase), and fats (lipase). They do all their work in the gastrointestinal tract and can help combat common issues such as indigestion, bloating, abdominal discomfort, and gas. I would not recommend using digestive enzymes for a prolonged time or on a daily basis; however, I did use them for a good few months myself when I was at the very beginning of my journey, and tried to decongest my system. They were helpful for some time, until my need for them naturally declined as my healing progressed and my body got detoxified.

Systemic enzymes help to build and maintain overall health. They may be taken to address specific issues, but are often used to promote prevention and provide general body support. Supported processes include the breakdown of excess mucus, fibrin, many toxins, allergens, and clotting factors. Many people use systemic enzymes instead of NSAIDS, or non-steroidal anti-inflammatory drugs, since they also can be helpful in the temporary reduction of swelling. Unlike NSAIDS, systemic enzymes are able to pinpoint only the harmful circulating immune complexes (CICs) without suppressing the CICs that are beneficial.

Systemic enzymes have also been found helpful for: fibrosis conditions caused by the hard, sticky protein called fibrin; reduction of scar tissue, also made up of fibrin; cleaning the blood of cellular waste and toxins, also supporting normal liver function; promoting immune system response by helping white blood cell efficiency; managing the overgrowth of yeast, and putting less stress on your liver.

Taken in combination with a healthy diet, supplements of digestive and systemic enzymes can help your body fight the effects of aging and improve your overall health.

I learned about this great supplement called "Beauty Enzymes" from David Wolfe, and I realized that I can expedite my body's detoxification by taking it. And because I was making my diet much lighter, I was concerned about my weight (I didn't want to lose it), so I thought it might help me with better absorption and prevent too much weight loss. Beauty Enzymes is a guaranteed plant-based supplement which is not irradiated, is free of genetically modified organisms (GMOs), and is grown to high specifications and purity requirements. This supplement is acid-resistant and remains active throughout the wide pH range found in the digestive system. Capsules contain bromelain and that are derived from controlled pineapple and papaya to ensure there is no risk of GMO contamination. I also learned that they put in some additives in most enzymes that are out on the market (for example, anti-caking agents that are toxic to us, or other unnecessary toxic stuff, like soybean oil). Beauty Enzymes don't have anything toxic in them, so I chose them over all other brands.

In addition to that, I learned that some enzymes can be systemic, and at the same time digestive. For example, if bromelain is taken with food, it will be assisting in digestion—and would therefore play a role of digestive enzyme. But, if you take it between meals (on empty stomach), it will act as a systemic enzyme: it will travel through your body finding unnecessary stuff, like extra protein that's settled on your arterial walls, and will help to dissolve all the toxic matter and goo that is stuck in you. Beauty Enzymes is both systemic and digestive: it can greatly assist with digestion. When taken on an empty stomach, Beauty Enzymes can have a more cleansing and detoxifying effect.

Why distilled water?

If you drink fruit and vegetable juices (freshly juiced), you are drinking distilled water plus certain nutrients such as fruit sugars, organic minerals and vitamins. But if you drink lake, river, or spring water, you are drinking undistilled water, plus all of the inorganic minerals that the water has picked up. This is known as hard water, meaning it has high inorganic mineral concentrations that can cause health problems.

Now, let's have a short lesson in chemistry. There are two kinds of chemicals: inorganic and organic. The inorganic chemicals are inert, which means that they can't be absorbed into the tissues of the body. Our bodies are composed of 16 organic minerals, all of which come from what is living or was once alive.

Organic minerals are very vital in keeping us alive and well. If we were cast away on an uninhabited island where nothing was growing, the regular person would starve to death. Even though the soil beneath our feet contains 16 inorganic minerals, our bodies could not absorb them. Only a living plant has the power to extract inorganic minerals from the earth. No human can extract the nourishment from inorganic minerals.

For years, people have said that certain waters were rich in all minerals. But were they talking about inorganic or organic minerals? Unfortunately, these are inorganic and these inert minerals are burdening our bodies, which may cause the development of stones in the kidneys, gallbladder and stone-like acid crystals in the arteries, veins, and other parts of the body.

Yet, you will hear people say: "Distilled water is dead water." But did you know that rain is distilled water? There are a lot of people who collect rainwater and use it for drinking, preparing food, and showering, and they appear to be the healthiest in comparison to people who don't drink distilled water. For example, if you go to the South Sea Islands, you will find an island inhabited by healthy

Polynesians who have never drank anything but distilled water, because the island is surrounded by the Pacific Ocean. Everyone knows that seawater is undrinkable, because of the high salt content. Their island is based on porous coral, which can't hold water, so they only have Mother Nature's distilled water to drink (i.e., rainwater and fresh coconut water). Several doctors thoroughly examined the oldest people on these islands, and they all concluded that they have never examined such well-preserved people in their lives. The older people looked much younger than their age as well, and they had a longer life span.

In the Navy, there are huge aircraft carriers with 5,000 Navy personnel aboard. These ships can't carry enough land water, so they distill seawater for the men to drink and bathe in. And big ocean cruise ships distill seawater for their passenger's use, bathing, etc. Yet, we haven't heard any complaints from any of the people that spent the lengthy times on the ships that they got sick due to drinking distilled water. There is no scientific evidence to support such a claim.

Distilled water helps to dissolve the terrible, toxic poisons that are collected in people's bodies. It passes through the kidneys without leaving inorganic pebbles and stones. If you wash your hair in rain (distilled) water, your hair will have extra softness. I personally don't have the equipment to distill my water, so I resort to the second-best option: RO water (Reverse Osmosis). This is the closest alternative that you can find to distilled water, and if you want to add "life" to your water, you can add few drops of freshly squeezed lemon, or cut few slices of fruit in your glass bottle of RO water. That will help to structure it and "bring your water to life" before you drink it.

The farther I go—the less I need

Before I started my journey, I used a lot of things that turned out to be unnecessary and detrimental to my health. For example, I used antiperspirant deodorant under my armpits that was blocking perspiration, which means that all the toxins didn't have a chance to exit with sweat and were trapped in my body. I was also using a lot of "skincare" products that our society encourages us to: cleansers, toners, lotions, serums, and body lotions. I used a lot of hair products: serums, conditioners, shining sprays, and hairsprays. I thought that all of those things didn't affect my health. I believed that by using all those products, I would prevent aging and maintain my body, skin, and hair at the top level. I was wrong. All of the stuff I used (and it was very expensive and trendy stuff) was purely toxic to my body.

Now, I am at the point where I detoxed enough that my hair don't require as much attention: I used to wash my hair every day (or sometimes every other day), because it would get greasy from all the toxic stuff I ate and put on top of my body. Now my hair doesn't get greasy as fast: I wash it only once a week, and it looks great. I have met people that are fruitarians for decades and they don't ever get greasy hair—they never use shampoo or conditioner, and only wash with water. I believe that I will eventually get there as well. I mentioned in an earlier chapter that I use only organic products. I also mentioned exactly what I use for my body, hair, teeth, and face. If you go over six months as a mono-fruitarian, it will happen to you as well.

I used to travel with six small bags stuffed with all those products that I thought I needed. Now I barely fill one small travel purse with all the things I need. Life became simpler. Less effort is involved in maintaining my skin, body, and hair—but the results are outstanding. I believe that we create the problems by ourselves, and then spend a lot of money on resolving them. For example, we eat toxic foods that cause us to break out and have acne all over, and then we spend a lot of money on finding that "magic pill" in a form of supplements, and creams, and lotions trying to fix the acne problem. Why not just stop eating all that "garbage" and have nice, clear, silky skin on its own, without ever spending a penny on "fixing the problem" that wouldn't have existed in the first place?

I always thought I understood the phrase, "We are what we eat," but I didn't really get the full meaning of it until I started experiencing all the benefits of being a fruitarian. Once my skin started looking 10 years younger, I realized that less truly is more. Within three years, my dark circles under my eyes were gone, any crow's feet around my eyes vanished, and my skin started to glow again, I started to understand the full meaning of how it is important not to use my body as a garbage can and mindlessly put everything I find tasty in my stomach.

Even more interesting, I started having grey hair. But after my diet transition, three years later, I couldn't find any grey hairs. They completely vanished—it was hard to believe! I would pull grey hairs out to inspect them, and see that at the root they would be totally dark ash blonde (my natural color): you could see a growth of at least of one inch of dark ash blond hair, and the end of the hair (another one inch or more) would be silver. I actually saved a few of these hairs as proof that it was real.

When it comes to food, it seems that I need to eat less with each passing month: I am getting full on two or three fruits a day. There are some days when I overeat, but that is done for the sake of flavor (followed by the discomfort of a full stomach until a few hours later, when the food is no longer in my stomach). The good part of being a fruitarian is that, even if you overeat, it doesn't last long. It takes an hour or so for it to go through. If you overeat on cooked and processed foods, you will feel stuffed for at least eight hours, and that is a lot of discomfort to go through, in my opinion.

Sometimes the idea of "to eat or not to eat" visits me. I feel like I don't need to eat any longer, but I do it out of boredom, so to speak, to "eat away" some kind of emotional state. In other cases, I'm eating for the experience of taste and flavor, and of course, out of habit. Believe me, you can enjoy the flavors of fresh organic fruits just as much as pizza (though fruits are not as addictive as pizza, they can be very charming sitting on the table as they lure you into eating them). Once, I was told: "Eat unless you have the reason not to..." Since then, I realized that some things are just a natural progression: you will change your lifestyle when you realize that you can't live by your old lifestyle habits. If I can't eat 2,000 calories (as society encourages), and if I am eating 200 or 400 calories a day (and only fruits), that means that this is all my body needs. If I feel at my optimal performance and health at 300 calories a day, then let it be—as long as you feel great and are not hurting yourself. There is no need to become anorexic or develop any other eating disorder. This book is not about that. There is no need to force yourself to do anything if you already feel great. I don't encourage you to starve yourself. All I encourage you is to make better food choices and never overeat just for the sake of enjoyment, or use eating as an escape from boredom. It is very important to listen closely to your body.

Every person is on his or her own journey of development. One person is trying to regain lost health, another is trying to fight acne or a life-threatening situation, another is trying to fix their greying hair, or some might use this lifestyle as a preventative measure for being able to sustain quality life for a longer period of time. No matter what the reason is, we are all on our journey to "better" ourselves. Just remember: each day we either progress in our goals, or regress. We don't stay still. And our actions of today will define our tomorrow— whether we get closer to our goal or farther away, it's all up to us.

How to start making

changes

During my journey from vegan to raw vegan, to fruitarian to mono-fruitarian, I learned that some things could be more useful if done at the beginning of transition.

For example, I would recommend using Colosan at the very beginning (this is the supplement for cleansing your intestines, discussed in an earlier chapter). When your intestines are congested from all-American cooked foods, it would be great to take a week and actually cleanse them. It won't cleanse your intestines 100%, as it takes much longer to remove all the build up from the intestinal walls, but it will help you to decongest them and give you a good start. I won't recommend using Colosan all the time; don't fall into the trap of thinking that you can take Colosan as a remedy each time you have processed foods. The general idea is to detox and cleanse. (And if you are a fruitarian, it is not necessary to take

Colosan—so you can completely omit this one.) The best intestinal detox is when you eat a mono-fruitarian diet for a month or two. The best choice would be grapes. The second would be watermelon.

I would highly recommend doing at least 10 sessions of colonics (preferably every other day) to cleanse out your large intestine from all the toxins that have accumulated there. It seems that people who just switched to vegan diet (not even fully raw) experience great benefits from it.

Once you have decongested your intestines (which shouldn't take you more then couple of weeks, but some professionals recommend stretching colonics sessions for a longer period of time), it's time to start gallstone flushes once a month. This will take you about a year or a little more than a year to completely flush your liver and gallbladder and remove all the stones. It is very important to be vegan (at the very least) once you start gallstone flushes, because otherwise it will be counterproductive: you will create new stones if you don't change your diet. On the other hand, you can omit gallstone flushes, and the stones can be dissolved on their own with the help of tinctures (see previous chapters). However, this approach might take a longer time to see results. The best option is a mono-fruitarian diet—it's a natural way of slowly dissolving the buildup in your system, including gallstones. Gallstone flushes are a short cut if you want to get rid of the toxic stones in your body faster. For me, one year of gallstone flushes made a huge difference in my health.

As part of your dietary transition, I would recommend to do it very slowly and gradually. I personally came across the difficulty of giving up my favorite childhood foods, and the comfort foods to which I was emotionally attached, because they were consumed around happy events and family gatherings. I had to choose healther substitutes for those foods, which was a real challenge at times. After research and a lot of trial and error, I realized that each step of the dietary transition could be an amazing experience of enjoying delicious, raw vegan dishes while progressing on a smooth (and even fun!) journey to ultimate health. I figured that it could be an exciting journey of exploration— not a chore to gain better health—while playing with flavors and foods, benefiting from each step of the transition.

There are some basic ideas that I think might be useful in your own dietary transition. Generally, I would not recommend anyone to go "cold turkey" and stop eating altogether. I wouldn't recommend anyone to go mono-fruitarian overnight either, because it might simply be dangerous for your health: you literally could drown from releasing too many of your own toxins into your system at once. It's a slow process of your body adjusting to incremental changes that you make, and you should have patience. It does take time to transition—but this is also what makes your journey fun, rather than a miserable, jolting detox trip that could put your own life or health at risk. Think of it this way: if you start making all changes at once, you are less likely to stick with it. But if you do one change at a time, and stick with it while enjoying the new flavors and experiences, then it could be an amazing and pleasant journey to ultimate health without any problems.

First, I would recommend eliminating all dairy (milk, cheese, yougurt, etc.) from your diet, as well as all animal products. Also, it would be great to learn how to substitute bread with healthier choices or eliminate it altogether. Don't try to go 100% raw right away. I think the task of eliminating dairy, animal products and breads, and to go 100% vegan is already a lot to handle from the get-go. Try to incorporate a diet of at least 50% raw foods; but most importantly, just make sure you can stick with eliminating dairy, animal products, and breads. Also, it is very important to learn how to substitute animal products with plant-based ones (for example, how to substitute cheese with a healthier, nut-based version). I would recommend sticking with this step for at least six months. Once you are adjusted to the changes, it is time to move forward.

For the second step, I would recommend going 100% raw vegan. You will be amazed at how diverse and flavorful raw vegan foods could be. Eating out might be a problem, so you have to be prepared to make your own food at home. If you "un-cook" at home in advance, it is hard to "fall off the wagon" once you already have a raw vegan version of pasta that is just as tasty or even better than the real thing. Raw vegan desserts taste better, in my opinion, than "regular" desserts. Like I said, the biggest problem with people transitioning into raw vegan foods is not knowing what can be prepared instead of cooked meals, because no one ever showed it to them. My father's response to me going 100% raw vegan was: "You can't survive on a couple of leaves of greens." And that's what people usually think when you say "raw vegan." But that's a huge misconception. Sure, there are a lot of greens involved in each recipe, but it could be extremely tasty and flavorful, and with varieties of different ingredients. You could have raw vegan "meatballs," "stuffed tacos," "pasta alfredo," "steak and mashed potatoes," "hash browns," "scrambled eggs," "waffles," and "chips." All of these foods resemble the real thing, yet they are even more flavorful, vibrant, and full of life. I would recommend staying raw vegan for at least six months to allow your body to fully adjust to changes.

The third step would be switching to a fruitarian diet. This is an amazing time when you get to experience all different fruits in abundance, and learn a variety of different recipes of how to make it work and still enjoy the food. Keep in mind, there are sweet and non-sweet fruits. For example, cucumber, avocado, tomato, and red bell pepper are all non-sweet fruits. You get to create a variety of awesome salads and desserts, and enjoy this stage of your dietary transition to the fullest. There are, of course some rules of how to properly combine fruits to heal your body. Without this knowledge, you can do more harm to your body than healing. It's all a matter of doing your homework and educating yourself.

And for optimal health, it would be best to finally transition to the fourth stage of a mono-fruitarian lifestyle. It is important to learn which fruits you can combine together and which should never be eaten at the same time. You should never eat just because it's lunchtime or dinner time. You should eat only when you feel hungry. At this stage, you will be fairly clean, and will have a very refined sense of smell and taste. And most importantly, you will be enjoying your optimal health: a lot of aging signs will disappear, and your resilience will shoot through the roof. You might need less sleep, and will not be getting tired as fast. Your energy will be endless, and you will be in a fantastic mood, always. It is very important to live not only a long life, but a high-quality life, and the fruitarian diet is proven to provide exactly this.

Regardless of where your journey leads you (it might be vegetarian, vegan, raw vegan, or fruitarian), I hope this book brought some light to why it's not beneficial to eat certain types of foods. I suggest trusting your own gut, and listening to your own body. It will always tell you what it needs (and please don't confuse those signals with mental cravings, like cooked pizza: there is nothing nutritious about it, it's just addictive and toxic). You can take your journey as far as you want to—don't be afraid to be adventurous! I wish you the best of health throughout this exciting exploration of better dietary choices and proper detoxing.

Made in the USA
Las Vegas, NV
12 December 2022

61988752R00360